F

SPEECH/LANGUAGE CLINICIAN'S HANDBOOK

SPEECH/LANGUAGE CLINICIAN'S HANDBOOK

Edited by

MAYNARD D. FILTER, Ph.D.

Department Head
Speech Pathology and Audiology
James Madison University
Harrisonburg, Virginia

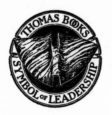

CHARLES C THOMAS · PUBLISHER
Springfield · Illinois · U.S.A.

Published and Distributed Throughout the World by
CHARLES C THOMAS • PUBLISHER
BANNERSTONE HOUSE
301-327 East Lawrence Avenue, Springfield, Illinois, U.S.A.

© *1979, by* CHARLES C THOMAS • PUBLISHER
ISBN 0-398-03899-6
Library of Congress Catalog Card Number: 78-31653

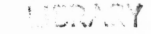
Printed in the United States of America
N-1

Library of Congress Cataloging in Publication Data

Main entry under title:

Filter
Speech/language clinician's handbook.

   Includes bibliographies and index.
   1. Speech, Disorders of—Handbooks, manuals, etc. 2. Speech disorders in children—Handbooks, manuals, etc. 3. Speech therapy—Handbooks, manuals, etc.
I. Filter, Maynard D.
RC423.S636   616.8'552   78-31653
ISBN 0-398-03899-6

CONTRIBUTORS

Julia R. Boxx, Ph.D., School of Communication Disorders, Cumberland College of Health Sciences, Haymarket New South Wales, Australia.

Mary Ellen Brandell, M.A., Division of Speech and Language Pathology, Communication Disorders, Central Michigan University, Mt. Pleasant, Michigan.

Maynard D. Filter, Ph.D., Department of Speech Pathology and Audiology, James Madison University, Harrisonburg, Virginia.

Leslie Gruber, Ph.D., Division of Speech and Language Pathology, Communication Disorders, Central Michigan University, Mt. Pleasant, Michigan.

Laura J. Kelly, M.A., Department of Audiology and Speech Science, Michigan State University, East Lansing, Michigan.

Sr. Marie A. Kopin, M.Sc., Division of Speech and Language Pathology, Communication Disorders, Central Michigan University, Mt. Pleasant, Michigan.

Connie Miller-Barnett, M.A., Carrollton Public Schools, Carrollton, Michigan.

Michael P. Rosenblatt, M.A., Minneapolis Otolaryngology, P.A., 363 Southdale Medical Building, 6545 France Avenue South, Edina, Minnesota.

Linda I. Seestedt, M.A., Division of Audiology, Communication Disorders, Central Michigan University, Mt. Pleasant, Michigan.

Marcia Weber-Olsen, Ph.D., Division of Speech and Language Pathology, Communication Disorders, Central Michigan University, Mt. Pleasant, Michigan.

PREFACE

THIS TEXT is designed specifically for the beginning clinician enrolled in a beginning clinical practicum experience in speech/language pathology. Each author was instructed to prepare a concise summary of approaches to assessment and remediation (if appropriate) of the specific area of which each has expertise, to minimize theoretical and etiological material found in abundance elsewhere, and to emphasize approaches to the clinical management of individuals with communicative disorders.

The main purposes of this book are to provide the speech/ language clinician with basic approaches to evaluation, assessment, and (re) habilitation of children and adults with communicative handicaps and to provide information on popular and modern (re) habilitative methods, procedures, and techniques. Our observations with both clinicians in training and clinicians in practice indicated that a basic text emphasizing evaluation and (re) habilitation was needed.

Many members of the Communication Disorders faculty at Central Michigan University volunteered to contribute a chapter in their area of expertise. After more than a year of labor, ten of the original group completed chapters. This text originated from an idea to provide a concise review of current methods for beginning practicum students at Central Michigan University; however, we believe that the information is appropriate for all beginning speech/language clinicians. The text also provides a concise review of modern approaches for the practicing clinician, especially those employed in the public schools.

M.D.F.

vii

ACKNOWLEDGMENTS

MANY INDIVIDUALS assisted in the development of this book. The patience, understanding, and assistance of our families, friends, colleagues, students, secretaries, and clients are acknowledged. A special acknowledgment to all our referenced colleagues from whom we borrowed many rich and innovative ideas which have helped us and will help others provide better speech and language services to the communicatively impaired.

The assistance of Beverly Ketchum in developing the chapter on articulation is acknowledged. The audiology figures were developed by Dennis Pompilius, graphic illustrator at Central Michigan University. Special thanks to my wife Judy and to my children Keith and Kellie for their patience and encouragement.

M.D.F.

CONTENTS

SPEECH/LANGUAGE
CLINICIAN'S HANDBOOK

Chapter 1

LANGUAGE ASSESSMENT IN CHILDREN: PRINCIPLES AND PERSPECTIVES

MARCIA WEBER-OLSEN

PROFESSIONALS interested in the remediation of childhood language disorders have been forced to keep pace with innumerable changes in child language research over the past decade. Perhaps the most pervasive of all these changes were efforts made by several linguists and psychologists in pioneering a discipline devoted to the study of language acquisition in children, e.g. Chomsky, 1965; Braine, 1963; Brown et al., 1964, 1968, 1973; McNeill, 1966, 1970; Slobin, 1970; Sinclair, 1971.

As a result of revolutionary changes made in the description of child grammars (Bloom, 1970; Brown, 1973; Bowerman, 1973), evaluative procedures for assessing delayed or deviant language skills in children have also undergone tremendous modification. Previous assessment approaches to the evaluation of childhood language disorders, e.g. Kirk, McCarthy, and Kirk, 1968, looked primarily at normative aspects of linguistic achievement in children rather than at the more individualistic and descriptive aspects of this behavior. Consequently, strategies and stylistic differences in children's approaches to language learning were at one time largely neglected in the evaluative process. Emphasis was placed on appraising the *products* rather than *processes* of language acquisition (Muma, 1978) so that children who did not manifest the appropriate "products" by a certain age or stage could be more readily diagnosed as linguistically deviant in some way. A child's language status was diagnostically classified as delayed, deviant, or even culturally disadvantaged relative to a set of statisti-

3

cal norms that did little more than identify whether a language problem did or did not exist (Muma, 1978).

Unfortunately, normative assessment data gave experienced diagnosticians very little edge over most beginning clinicians in exploiting possible clinical alternatives with populations of communicatively handicapped children (Muma, 1978). Other than naming skills, color and object sorting, and a few other rudimentary discrimination and categorization skills, many speech clinicians were (and regretfully, still are) at a loss to know what more significant aspects of the child's linguistic behavior required intervention.

Even if some continuity between diagnostic and therapeutic settings is aspired to, professionals are still plagued with finding ways to remediate deficit linguistic skills identified in children's evaluation reports. Too often, evaluative procedures become superfluous when information gained from assessment is disregarded because clinicians know of no way to operationalize this information in therapeutic ways or because this information has little relevance to any of the prepackaged language training programs that are currently in use. Fortunately, advances in child language research have begun to rectify these clinical problems and have provided some resolution of difficult clinical decisions that await all language clinicians at some point in their professional experience.

The following discussion will examine an approach to language assessment that reflects more recent developmental perspectives in child language acquisition and ways of implementing the changes suggested by this corpora of research. Not all aspects of the diagnostic process nor the linguistic capacities of all types of language delayed children will be exhaustively reviewed, but several fundamentals of language assessment will be developed in the hope that more comprehensive evaluative undertakings can build on the framework presented in this chapter.

A basic overview of the diagnostic process will be undertaken first so that any later discussion of language assessment can be integrated within this evaluative framework. A more comprehensive look at several available test instruments and procedures for assessing language skills will be presented next, followed by a brief discussion about related aspects of language development including cognition.

An Evaluative Framework

Speech or language assessment involves a series of evaluative steps taken by a diagnostician to determine the communicative status of an individual. In the field of language disorders, a comprehensive description of the communicative, cognitive, and socio-affective status of the child is ultimately of concern to the speech clinician and has been traditionally upheld as the primary purpose of the initial or final evaluation. Therapeutic endeavors originate and culminate with assessment and are shaped by diagnostic decisions made at strategic points in the clinical process. It is understandable, then, that two critical questions facing many beginning clinicians involve the *when* and *how* of assessment: what is the best timetable for evaluating a client's communicative status? Once this decision is reached, it is then desirable to have a definite strategy or plan of action for operationalizing the assessment schedule. Figure 1-1 illustrates this evaluative framework in more detail; it schematizes basic *when* and *how* steps and decisions that face the speech and language diagnostician. The model is arranged hierarchically to delineate chronological orders of these events and how they inter-relate in the assessment process.

Few clinicians still find advantages with older pre– post assessment approaches that chronologically restrict evaluation modes to periods immediately preceding and following therapy. An assessment mode that makes these kinds of modifications only "after the fact," i.e. at the conclusion of an extensive therapeutic period, will miss capitalizing on those benefits that can be derived from more recent evaluative information. Current approaches to the evaluation and remediation of language disabilities instead strongly advocate an ongoing means of assessment, e.g. Stremel and Waryas, 1974; Miller and Yoder, 1974; Bricker, Ruder, and Vincent-Smith, 1976; Guess, Sailor, and Baer, 1974. Such a strategy allows for continual re-evaluation of therapeutic effectiveness and accommodates the content and teaching strategies of a language program to the constantly changing communicative needs of the child.

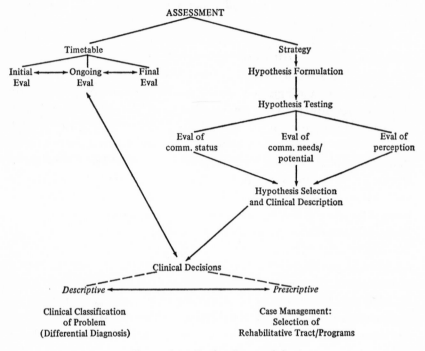

Figure 1-1. Evaluation model.

Although assessment maximally serves the needs of the client when it is ongoing, this does not weaken the primary value of the initial evaluation report in providing a detailed description and probable clinical diagnosis of a client's communication problem immediately prior to the onset of therapy. The initial evaluation provides a starting point and frame of reference for later evaluation and therapy, so it is important that a strategy or plan of action for carrying out this first stage of assessment be clarified *before* the clinician begins the evaluation. Nevertheless, the how-to-go-about-it aspect of clinical assessment is perhaps one of the most anxiety-invoking situations for many beginning speech clinicians. Guided more by routine than by a clinical rationale, many students make the mistake of plunging headlong into a speech or language evaluation with a battery of tests, which they compulsively administer regardless of the client's problem or complaint. The unfortunate consequences of this situation are too often apparent: an overly tested client who eventually refrains from displaying his maximum test performance out of boredom, fatigue, or frustration with the test situation and a confused clinician who must decipher a haphazard and often conflicting set of test results. Schultz (1973) has discussed other disadvantages of this type of assessment strategy, referring to it as a "post hoc" method of evaluation in which a clinician "typically uses all of a pre-established set of tests and subsequently scores, analyzes and synthesizes the results" to come to various diagnostic decisions about the client. An "on-line" mode of assessment, in contrast to post hoc evaluation procedures, avoids arbitrary and unguided pre-selection of test instruments since it involves "running analyses which terminate when the clinician is satisfied she has reached her goal."

How does the speech clinician systematically evaluate a client's complaint or problem? Ultimately, the clinician's goal or strategy is to eliminate or reduce his/her uncertainty about the client's communicative status (Schultz, 1973). Initial intake information obtained from case histories and/or interviews with the client or his caretakers often directs the clinician to consider several alternative explanations and possible etiologies (causes) about the client's disorder or complaint of which only one or a combination will best resolve the clinician's uncertainty. Development of alternative explanations during initial assessment is thus analogous to the *formulation* and subsequent testing of several statistical hypotheses. Statistical hypotheses predict various empirical outcomes that can be generalized to a larger population of observations. Clinical hypotheses as defined here are tentative statements that predict different *communicative* outcomes (Schultz, 1973). Hypotheses are *tested* through observation and formal assessment of the client's perceptual, motor, and verbal behavior. These resulting data, in turn, resolve the "truth" or "falsity" of previously formulated hypotheses and guide the final *selection* of a hypothesis that conforms best to the client's test performance and overall profile of communicative abilities.

Medical, social, and other psychological factors also have a key role in determining which of these hypotheses is more likely than others and which ones can be confidently eliminated. Clinicians who hope to systematically eliminate certain hypotheses while maximizing others must not only account for these kinds of factors but must also select test instruments that adequately discriminate the hypotheses they wish to test (Schultz, 1973; Schultz and Carpenter, 1974). Even before test selection, clinicians must decide the plausibility of their hypotheses and assign probabilities to these statements so that only the most likely diagnostic explanations are entertained during assessment (Schultz, 1973). Schultz (1973) has compared assessment procedures such as these to a two-step induction-deduction process: induction involves collecting and processing "sufficient material to formulate a set of hypotheses that are reasonable and are likely to contain the 'true' hypothesis." Deduction entails selection of material that will discriminate alternative hypotheses "with the goal of eliminating all but one."

Once a single hypothesis is found that best fits and explains the evaluative data (outcomes) at hand, the clinician is in a better position to describe and/or diagnose the client's communicative problem. Although differential diagnosis is one objective of the assessment process, it is not always easily fulfilled and may await the development of more sensitive assessment procedures or instruments.

Clinical diagnosis, hence, is not an inevitable outcome of initial assessment although *clinical description* of the problem is. In either event, both description and diagnosis require the diagnostician to put his appraisal of the client in context. The speech clinician must integrate all relevant information on the background and current status of the client (Emerick and Hatten, 1974), including knowledge about factors contributing to and maintaining the individual's communicative problem if a problem does, in fact, exist. The clinician uses this information to come to clinical decisions about the nature and severity of a communication disorder and the client's potential for changing or improving his communicative status.

Assessment, therefore, takes on a twofold purpose that is both *descriptive* and *prescriptive* in its aim. Clinical descriptions and classifications of the type, nature, and severity of a problem guide clinical decisions for selecting rehabilitative programs matched to the problem. Prognostic statements, which predict the probabilities and conditions for achieving "communicative normalcy," direct remedial programs by specifiying the client's most urgent communicative needs and his willingness and potential for change (Schultz and Carpenter, 1974). Attitudinal factors, hence, play a critical role in the assessment process since they guide the selection of a therapy model suited to the client's own perceptions of his problem.

Beginning clinicians can be more thorough in their evaluative endeavors by examining not only their self-formulated hypotheses about the client but the opinions of the client as well; for example, whether the client considers his present communicative status a problem (it is often the clinician's duty to counsel those individuals who wrongly perceive that a communicative problem exists), whether he feels that therapy is a necessary step to correcting this problem, whether he will be committed to this decision once enrolled in rehabilitation, and so on.

Since the costs of receiving therapeutic services for a communication problem often far outweigh the values, it is the clinician's role to advise the client to carefully consider these assets and liabilities and the client's potential for suceeding. A laryngectomee, for example, may be very willing to master esophageal speech, but the success of his efforts toward achieving this goal are largely dependent on whether he can adequately inject air into the esophagus. The clinician, then, must direct the client to objectively consider these potential risks and to consider the best alternatives for dealing with his communication situation. Beginning clinicians can shape these decisions by carefully examining motivational factors as well as pertinent behavioral variables in the communicatively handicapped.

In summary, an evaluative framework has been adopted for discussion, which considers the *when* and *how* of assessment, i.e. a recommended *timetable* for conducting evaluations and a logical *strategy* for initiating assessment. It was mentioned that an assessment mode that is ongoing in nature is more responsive to the changing communicative needs of the client. Clinical procedures that build in evaluations at successive periods throughout therapy have largely replaced outmoded clinical approaches that evaluate only in a pre–post mode, i.e. immediately prior to and following the remediation period.   Assessment, in general, involves the formulation and "online" testing of several hypotheses that render the evaluation process more efficient and concomitantly reduce uncertainty about the client's communicative status.

Clinical hypotheses are tentative statements that predict different communicative outcomes.   Hypotheses are differentially weighted in terms of their likelihood in correctly predicting a client's communicative status.   Clinicians are encouraged to systematically select test instruments and assessment procedures that will discriminate among these hypotheses.   Certain hypotheses will be eliminated and others maximized based on a client's test performance. Hence, the systematic selection of test instruments and procedures aids in the resolution of a clinical hypothesis that best predicts the client's behavior.

Hypothesis formulation and testing ultimately guide clinical decisions during assessment.   These decisions may be either descriptive, e.g. assigning a client to a diagnostic category, or prescriptive in nature, e.g. selecting a rehabilitation tract that is suitable to the communicative needs and potential of the client.

Finally, it was mentioned that assessment of attitudinal factors in the communicatively handicapped assists in the selection of a therapy model individualized to the client's communicative needs and his perception of those needs.   This discussion will attempt to actualize these assessment steps, including the formulation, testing, and selection of hypotheses, with an exemplary clinical case further on in the chapter.

A Developmental Approach to Language Assessment

Graham (1976) and Ruder and Weber-Olsen (in press) have reviewed much of the recent child language intervention research that aligns with one of two major models of language acquisition: (1) a developmental model that adheres to normal language acquisition data and psycholinguistic research (Stremel and Waryas, 1974; Bricker and Bricker, 1974; Miller and Yoder, 1974) and (2) a nondevelopmental approach based primarily on behavior theory, which does not utilize normal acquisition data for determining the *content* and *sequence* of a language intervention program (Guess, Sailor, and Baer, 1974; Gray and Ryan, 1973; Carrier, 1974). Ruder and Weber-Olsen have highlighted the assets and limitations of both types of intervention approaches for different populations of language deviant children but endorse the developmental approach as a more desirable intervention strategy.

Psycholinguistic orientations to language training have stipulated that child language approximates a rule-bound system unique from adult rules of grammar (Bricker, Ruder, and Vincent-Smith, 1976; Waryas and Stremel-Campbell, in press). Hence, the frequency of grammatical forms and constructions and their usual orders of emergence in child speech serve as important milestones hallmarking normal language development. Sets of linguistic skills are considered prerequisites to succeeding stages of language development; deficits in one or any number of these skills might predict whether a child is deviating too far from the normal developmental sequence and, therefore, is a suitable candidate for language intervention.

Indeed, there is some evidence to document that many language deviant children follow the normal language acquisition sequence but merely at a slower rate than normal children (Johnston and Schery, 1976; Lackner, 1968; Morehead and Ingram, 1973). Johnston and Schery compared the acquisition of eight grammatical morphemes in 287 language deviant children representing different linguistic levels of development. Their data closely approximated acquisitional data for normal children (Brown, 1973; DeVilliers and DeVilliers, 1973) and suggested that the language deviant child proceeds through an invariant acquisition order but at a markedly slower rate than the normal child. Developmental orders of emergence have been carefully blueprinted by language interventionists who hope to develop a series of discrete training steps that lead the language delayed child from early grammatical forms to developmentally later forms.

Although developmental models of language acquisition have helped tremendously in the identification and remediation of language handicapped children, these procedures are far from being conventionalized since research surprisingly indicates that emergence patterns for several grammatical structures are not altogether invariant in their sequence (Bloom, 1970; Bloom, Hood, and Lightbown, 1975; Nelson, 1973; Braine, 1976). Important differences in individual cognitive styles and language input factors are often obscured by the overwhelming number of language similarities across children. Nevertheless, these differences do suggest that more than one major developmental sequence may exist and await further empirical confirmation in normal children who display it in their linguistic development.

Comparative assessment of language skills in normal and language delayed children, therefore, may not be an entirely reliable undertaking depending on the vulnerability of current psycholinguistic research to disproof. The following discussion will consider several parameters of linguistic development and ways of assessing these parameters with this precautionary note in mind. For reasons already put forward, a developmental model of language acquisition will be adopted for discussion.

Four parameters of linguistic development, including phonological, morphological, syntactical, and semantic aspects, will be briefly defined for later inclusion in the chapter. Next we will consider a few of the advantages and disadvantages that are inherent to formal versus informal measures of language assessment, followed by a more comprehensive discussion of the two major response modalities of language: comprehension and production. The discussion will attempt to interrelate these two response modalities with the four major linguistic parameters mentioned above as several formal language measures and other informal evaluation procedures are reviewed. Ways in which these measures can be used for solving different clinical hypotheses will be considered.

In the final portion of this chapter, the evaluation of some communicative and cognitive skills that are germaine to the child's language development will be briefly examined.

The Parameters of Linguistic Development
Phonology
A phoneme has been defined as the smallest unit of speech that makes a difference linguistically (Winitz, 1969). Thus,

phonemes distinguish words such as *bad* vs. *pad, pet* vs. *pat* that are topographically similar in composition but signal altogether different meanings in the language.

Speech clinicians use a variety of available articulation test instruments (Goldman and Fristoe, 1969; Templin and Darley, 1969) to assess the child's mastery of phoneme production in the language (see Chapter 5 of this volume for a more comprehensive description on articulation assessment). It is unfortunate that many beginning clinicians choose to neglect concomitant language deficits in those children who display deviant phonological development merely because the evaluation and treatment of articulation disorders have earned separate clinical status from the treatment of other communicative disorders. On the contrary, a great deal of phonological research has successfully countered the once traditional assumption that articulation and language are functionally independent mechanisms. Age-inappropriate misarticulations in children frequently correlate with language deficits in the same population reflecting various morphological deviations (Templin, 1969) syntactical deficits (Menyuk, 1964; Menyuk and Looney, 1972; Shriner, Holloway, and Daniloff, 1969), and semantic deviations (Menyuk and Looney, 1972) in children's production of language. These findings have led researchers to recommend broadly based language training programs over traditional single-phoneme approaches for simultaneously improving both articulation and grammatical skills in children.

Though a causal relationship between grammatical and phonological processes is yet to be further substantiated, current research admonishes that phonological skills should not be evaluated out of context within a broader language framework. Remediation of articulation deficits otherwise becomes a nearsighted and unnecessarily time-consuming task that loses relevance to the total communicative needs of the language handicapped child.

Morphology

Morphemes can be defined as the smallest meaningful units of the language. Thus morphology deals with the study of morphemes and the ways in which they are arranged and structurally combine with each other in the language (MacLeish, 1971). Morphemes can stand alone at *free morphemes* in the language to signal different meanings or combine with other morphemes. Morphemes that cannot stand alone in the language but have combinatorial power are *bound morphemes;* they create structural variations in a word, which modulate its original meaning in certain predictable ways.   The free morpheme *boy,* for example, cannot be broken down into any smaller meaningful units in the language.   When *boy* becomes *boys* by addition of the bound plural morpheme [–s], its meaning now signals something slightly different.   Similarly, the bound [–s] morpheme when added to the word *top* will predictably change its meaning from singular *(top)* to plural *(tops).*

Children's spontaneous production of bound and free morphemes in the language can be used as an index of their general stage of linguistic development.   Other indices, such as chronological age, are generally an unsatisfactory indicator of a young child's linguistic sophistication (Brown, 1973).   By computing the average frequency of morphemes in a child's speech, that is his mean number of morphemes per utterance (mean length of utterance), clinicians can get a fairly reliable estimate of a child's language development.

The following section of this chapter will devote discussion to the assessment of morphological skills in children, including mean length of utterance (MLU) measures.

Syntax

Syntax has been traditionally defined as that aspect of linguistic development that involves rules of word order.   In child language acquisition, syntactical development reflects not only the child's knowledge of word order, i.e. how elements are arranged in a sentence, but also the functional relationships of these elements (Bowerman, 1975).   Syntactic relationships dictate how words combine in a sentence to result in lawful grammatical sequences.   The words *daddy* and *pushed,* for example, can be arranged in two ways; if the noun *daddy* precedes *pushed* in a sentence, such as *"Daddy pushed* the lawnmower," the two words designate a subject-predicate syntactic relationship. When *pushed* precedes *daddy* in the sentence, "I *pushed daddy*," the syntactic relationship now changes from subject-predicate to a verb–direct object relationship. Language handicapped children often lack knowledge of the various rules that order words in the language, so their speech is often ungrammatical and syntactically deviant, e.g. "Mom store go this afternoon." A number of language tests attempt to carefully assess those syntactical rules that are deficient in the child through both production and comprehension response modes. These will be discussed at length in the next section.

Semantics

The study of semantic development involves the acquisition of meanings that various classes of words serve and the meaningful relationships into which they can enter. Semantics also deals with a description of individual word meanings, i.e. referential meanings. A child's referential word use reflects his vocabulary or lexical skills. Lexical meanings, in turn, have been used interchangeably to designate referential meanings; they reflect dictionary type of definitions for nouns, verbs, adjectives, and adverbs that signal concrete notions in the language (MacLeish, 1971). However, when words in combination with each other serve different semantic functions or relationships, we are concerned with their *combinatorial* meanings.

The assessment of semantic skills in the child examines how children arrange words in an utterance to produce different combinatorial meanings or semantic intentions in the language.

Nevertheless, it is exceedingly difficult to represent a child's semantic knowledge without careful consideration of the *communicative context* that surrounds a child's utterances. A normal two year old's utterance, "Mommy sock," therefore, could have two possible semantic interpretations: elaborated as "Mommy is putting on my sock" or "This is Mommy's sock." It would be impossible to determine which of these two meanings was actually *intended* by the child without sufficient knowledge of the child's immediate communicative environment, e.g. persons or objects present in the room; ongoing or past activities of the day, etc.

Documentation of these types of nonlinguistic settings is necessary if the child's intended meaning for "Mommy sock" is to be reliably disambiguated from other plausible semantic interpretations.

Several semantic functions and relationships, which normal children characteristically display throughout their language development, and assessment measures that evaluate these skills in the language deficient child will be considered.

Informal vs. Formal Language Assessment

An overwhelmingly large number of standardized language tests are available for formal language assessment purposes. A standardized test traditionally summarizes a child's overall performance relative to the expected performance, i.e. normative data. Typical age group performance is, in turn, determined relative to the repeated performance of a large number of children who are individually administered the test under identical test conditions. Thus, formal assessment procedures have the advantage of identifying a child's normative performance; tests falling into this category have been systematically developed and tested on many children to determine if a single child's performance coincides with or deviates from a statistically derived *performance average.* Children who deviate statistically far enough from this average (or norm) may be either accelerated or delayed in their development. Most formal language assessment measures are sensitive to finding children who fall in the latter category.

A good number of formal language measures profile a child's individual deficits (problem areas) by examining performance across several parameters of linguistic development and pinpointing the child's errors on each. However, a majority of formal language measures do not analyze or account for behavioral strategies that may have led to a correct or incorrect response; instead these tests usually serve to summarize the child's overall performance. Clinicians who rely heavily on evaluative information gathered from formal tests probably realize the benefits of using other *informal* assessment procedures as well. The majority of informal language measures are clinician-constructed and, therefore, serve a useful purpose in detailing the specific nature of a child's difficulty on a language task. Informal measures can be used to probe many more of the same language structures that were sampled on a formal language test. Materials and stimuli can be designed so that they systematically test a child's strategies. For example, it may be desirable to know why a child could not discriminate a sentence such as "The man kicks chair" from "The lady kicks the man." Since only certain grammatical elements vary across these two sentences, a clinician might then decide to directly probe whether the child knew the grammatical functions of subject and direct object in the language. Tasks requiring picture discrimination have been used quite successfully to assess children's comprehension of various grammatical elements in a sentence, including grammatical relations such as those mentioned above. Fraser, Bellugi, and Brown (1963), for example, constructed pairs of stimulus pictures so that they varied along only one grammatical dimension to test children's knowledge of contrastive sentences, such as "The mommy kisses the daddy" vs. "The daddy kisses the mommy." In this example, both subject and direct object constructions are being tested in the same sentence because the reversible sentence elements permit it.

Similarly, if a clinician desired a way of informally assessing a child's comprehension of various prepositions, such as *in, on, out,* and *off,* the clinician might select linguistic features that minimally contrasted the prepositional meanings and let this guide the selection of various objects that would permit equiprobable response alternatives for all four of these spatial relationships. Thus, the probability of a child demonstrating an *out* or *off* action should be equal in the same task and across all tasks in the informal assessment procedure. In this way, the clinician maintains control over those features he/she desires to vary and those he/she desires to keep constant (in this example, objects remain constant while spatial relationships vary), as well as other behavioral strategies, e.g. object or action preferences, that might otherwise disguise a child's actual knowledge of the language.

Informal assessment procedures have certain advantages over formal tests of language since the former attempt to identify the source of a child's language difficulties; these might entail, for example, inattention to rules of word order in the language or inability to assign words to various grammatical classes (nouns, verbs, adjectives, etc.). Informal tasks tell what a child can do under certain manipulative conditions; they often sample many more of the same language structures that were discovered to be deficient on previously administered formal test measures in order to look more comprehensively at the strategies a language handicapped child may use in comprehending and producing language. The obvious disadvantage is the inability of most informal measures to comment in any way on the child's performance relative to his own peer group. Informal measures, therefore, are restricted to individual assessment; comparative peer-performance statements are not possible unless normative data on a particular language task have been established for a reasonably large group of children.

Evaluating the Modalities of Language: Tests of Comprehension and Production

Many language clinicians were familiar with the terms *comprehension* and *production* long before Fraser, Bellugi, and Brown (1963) popularized their putative functional relationships in the normal language acquisition process. For purposes of this discussion, comprehension can be generally defined as understanding of the spoken message; it reflects *receptive* processes in the speaker-listener. Production, on the other hand, involves a speaker-listener's self-generated linguistic message and, therefore, reflects expressive processes. Speech represents the most common production modality, but alternate sensorimotor modalities can also be invoked for production of a linguistic message, for example, either graphically in written symbols, manually in signs, or even through different arrangements of arbitrarily shaped plastic symbols that have some communicative value between speaker and listener. The latter communicative system has been used quite successfully in establishing a rudimentary linguistic repetoire in the chimpanzee (Premack, 1971; Rumbaugh, 1977).

Decoding and encoding are terms often used interchangeably with comprehension and production. Decoding involves reception of a linguistic signal (input) as well as cognitive analysis and organization of this message, resulting in some recognition of its meaning. Encoding involves generation of a linguistic message (output) much like the print-out of a complex and intricately programmed computer system; integrated processes are at work in both the decoding and encoding of a linguistic message. Hence, these terms will be used at certain points throughout the chapter to more accurately specify the actual *mechanics* of comprehension and production.

Diagnosticians and clinicians are probably well aware of the debate over the developmental emergence of particular comprehension and production abilities in children (cf. Ingram, 1974, for a review of the issues). Although the traditional assumption has been that understanding (comprehension) must precede use (production) of the language, there is a growing body of evidence documenting that this relationship does not always hold for the acquisition of certain language structures (Chapman and Miller, 1974; Bloom, 1974; Keeney and Wolfe, 1972). Although the issues revolving around this strongly contested subject will not be brought into this discussion, it is perhaps best to acknowledge Bloom's (1974) view that asymmetries or developmental gaps in the receptive versus productive abilities of the normal child may reflect variable shifts in their influence on normal language development. Thus, it is extremely important for the beginning clinician to keep in mind not only the primary modality in which a particular assessment tool measures language but *also* possible explanations for any asymmetries in receptive vs. expressive abilities in the language delayed.

Clinical hypotheses can often be easily resolved by selecting tests and instruments that reveal whether a receptive-expressive gap exists or whether receptive and expressive language skills are roughly equivalent in the language handicapped child. Diagnostic information of this type will be quite useful in selecting a rehabilitative program suited to the child's communicative needs. If, for example, the child already displays adequate comprehension of certain grammatical structures but does not use these structures age-appropriately in his productive speech, then clinicians should consider intervention routes that bypass traditional receptive training steps in favor of intensive training in a production response mode (cf. Stremel and Waryas, 1974, for an exemplary intervention program) .

Some language intervention approaches have developed intricate nonverbal, i.e. receptive, systems of communication as a means of *initiating* the nonverbal, severely language delayed child into the language process so the transition to programs requiring speech as the primary response mode will be somewhat less difficult, e.g. Carrier, 1974; 1976. In the following section it will be helpful for the reader to individually list the receptive-expressive abilities that each language test and/or procedure evaluates.

Language assessment will vary dramatically from one child to the next, so very few of the techniques mentioned here can be viewed as routine steps for every language evaluation. It was recommended earlier in this chapter that efficiency in the assessment process was to be gained through formulation and systematic testing of clinical hypotheses about the client's communicative status, so the actual assessment of language disabilities in children will be approached from this same perspective. What we desire is a "narrowing down" of a range of plausible hypotheses rather than haphazard and unnecessary testing that will confound the overall clinical "picture" of the child. Our aim is to eliminate hypotheses that do not fit this picture as efficiently as possible without being redundant, i.e. administering tests that measure identical sets of skills or overlap excessively in skill assessment, and without sacrificing important diagnostic information by neglecting to be comprehensive enough in our search.

Figure 1-2 illustrates one approach to a systematic assessment of several language skills discussed previously in this chapter. If deficits are suspected in one or several of these skill areas, a sample of formal and informal language measures that will lead to the best resolution of our original hypothesis should be selected. If, for example, a case history form and parent interview initially profiled a child as "extremely difficult to understand, unable to produce most speech sounds, displaying a three-word intelligible vocabulary, unable to respond orally in the classroom but responsive to other's speech and capable of following instructions and directives at home and school," a plausible hypothesis might be that this child's articulation and expressive language skills will be age-inappropriate and depressed relative to her language comprehension skills. Formal and informal tests that maximize this hypothesis and eliminate other, less likely hypotheses, e.g. expressive and receptive skills will be equably depressed, can then be systematically selected. Some form of *receptive* lexical skill assessment would be justified for this child since her limited and unintelligible expressive vocabulary is probably one manifestation of her severe articulation difficulties. Therefore, we want to select other language measures that will optimize this child's receptive performance while avoiding tests that unfairly tax her expressive channels of communication.

The Peabody Picture Vocabulary Test (PPVT) (Dunn, 1959) or Ammons Full Range Vocabulary Test (Ammons and Ammons, 1977) would be appropriate for assessing this child's receptive lexical repetoire since both require picture recognition of several nouns, verbs, adjectives, and adverbs. The PPVT arranges vocabulary items in a developmental sequence so their referential meanings increase in semantic abstractness. Items are represented by a series of picture test plates with three decoy pictures and the target picture appearing on the same page. The young child is

Nature of Linguistic Skills				
Lexical		*FORMAL MEASURES*		*INFORMAL MEASURES*
	PPVT	(C*)		
Morpho-logical	AMMONS	(C)		
	Carrow TALC	(C)	DSS/DST	Berko's (1958) Morphological Test (P)
	ITPA-GRAM Closure	(C)	MLU (P)	
			Lang Analysis (P)	
Syntactic-Semantic	NSST	(C & P)	ELI (P)	Fraser *et al.'s* (1963) ICP Tasks (C & P)
	Carrow TALC	(C)	DSS/DST (P)	Preference Procedure (C)
	ACLC	(C)	Lang Analysis (P)	Hoduns (1975) Reinforced Search Task (C)

*C and P designate measures of *comprehension* and *production* respectively.

Figure 1-2. An assessment approach.

instructed to identify each target vocabulary item (spoken by the examiner) using a pointing response. Thus, the PPVT assesses vocabulary in a receptive mode and requires a nonverbal response from the child that is topologically simply and straightforward.

Once we have determined this child's lexical status and have judged her ability to perform in a nonverbal response mode with relatively easy to follow test instructions, we can select additional measures that are best suited to this child's communicative level and that will also clarify the hypothesis further. If this child were unable to attend to the PPVT stimulus materials, could not make the appropriate pointing response, or displayed other perceptual difficulties, for example, in not being able to visually discriminate pictures represented on each test plate, we may want to consider several makeshift, informal language measures as an alternative assessment procedure. If this child displayed no unusual test-taking difficulties with the PPVT, we might proceed with other formal assessment measures until we had satisfactorily proven or disproven our hypotheses or (depending on our assessment objectives) had alternately sampled and chosen one of several language rehabilitative tracts for this child.

A very common test profile in language assessment is a child who displays age-appropriate lexical skills (as determined by a vocabulary measuring device) but whose conversational speech is, nevertheless, grammatically aberrant in some way. It is helpful in these evaluative situations to recall that a child's knowledge of individual words and their referential meanings in the language differs from his knowledge about the semantic-syntactic relationships of words and their various combinatorial meanings. Several other assessment instruments more specifically measure this latter type of linguistic knowledge. The Carrow Test of Auditory Comprehension of Language (TALC) (Carrow, 1973) and the Assessment of Children's Language Comprehension Test (ACLC) (Foster, Giddan, and Stark, 1972) are two formal measures that systematically evaluate a child's comprehension of single lexical items that appear later in various morphological and/or syntactical constructions in the same test. In this way, clinicians are assured that a child who incorrectly comprehends "ball under the table" does so not because he lacks understanding of the referential meanings of these words but because he incorrectly processes the grammatical relationships that hold between the individual elements in this sentence.

A number of other formal and informal language measures, such as the Northwestern Syntax Screening Test (NSST) (Lee, 1969), the Elicited Language Inventory (Carrow, 1974), and the imitation, comprehension, and production tasks devised by Fraser et al. (1963), lack this inherent test feature. Nevertheless, the NSST has the advantage of assessing a child's comprehension and production of comparable grammatical structures. This test contains twenty stimulus sentence pairs that reflect grammatical contrasts varying in syntactic-semantic complexity. The construction of the NSST replicated the informal comprehension and production task devised by Fraser et al. (1963). In the receptive task, sentence pairs that contrast only one syntactic element are represented by a pair of stimulus pictures, which the child must identify by pointing to each picture in succession. Two other decoy pictures are included on the same test plate to minimize the probability of guessing. The Carrow TALC and the ACLC also have picture test plates that contrast target grammatical structures with decoy pictures deviating slightly from the target picture, e.g. a car bumping a train versus a train bumping a car. Thus, these measures all have ways of analyzing the child's errors in terms of their semantic-syntactic similarity to the target stimulus.

The expressive portion of the NSST employs a delayed imitation procedure in assessing the child's production of contrastive sentence pairs. Two pictures are represented on each test plate, corresponding to each stimulus sentence pair; the examiner verbally models each stimulus sentence for the child, then points to each picture in succession and elicits a delayed imitative response from the child, requesting him to "Tell me about this picture." Scoring instructions stipulate that the child must reproduce sentences in identical grammatical form to receive full credit on both. Although research has established the overall reliability and validity of the NSST (Ratusnik and Koenigsknecht, 1975), a study by Prutting, Gallagher, and Mulac (1975) found that 30 percent of the syntactical structures produced incorrectly on the expressive portion of this test by twelve language deviant children were used appropriately in the children's spontaneous speech. These latter authors recommend that the NSSTs expressive subtest cannot be used as a valid comprehensive assessment of spontaneous syntactical skills in the language delayed child but merely as a screening device. The beginning clinician who is aware of certain limitations of a formal language test such as the NSST and can select other formal and informal measures to compensate for these shortcomings will ultimately be more confident in the final hypothesis selection and evaluative descriptions of the child.

Imitation procedures obviously give us only a small insight into the child's productive and spontaneous use of the language, but comprehension procedures have their restrictions as well. Waryas and Ruder (1974) have criticized the traditional picture recognition format of most language comprehension tests for failing to determine "fine contrasts between grammatical and ungrammatical forms in order to determine whether the child knows when a given rule must or must not apply." A child who is asked to identify "the boy is running" versus "the boys are running" could be decoding each sentence on the basis of two co-occurring cues, i.e. whether the noun was singular or plural *or* whether the auxilliary verb was represented as *is* or *are* in the sentence. Hence, we have no assurance that the child demonstrates full comprehension of the grammatical rules governing subject-verb agreement since reliance on *either* of the two strategies above could lead the child to a correct response.

To alleviate these inherent difficulties in comprehension assessment, Waryas and Ruder devised a *procedure* in which the child was presented with a single visual test plate and two prerecorded (audio) stimuli and was requested to select the better (audio) match to the picture. In this respect, children's grammatical organization of various co-occurring rules in the language could be systematically tapped by testing their *preference* in judging stimulus sentences as more or less appropriate for a given picture.

Similarly, a *reinforced search procedure* was developed by Hodun (1975) to arrive at a more accurate assessment of normal children's comprehension of different spatial prepositions.

Hodun's contention is that the use of particular stimulus objects often invites certain object or action preferences in children that can disguise their actual knowledge about spatial terms in the language. For example, younger children prefer putting things *inside* something else rather than *on* or *under* whenever the referent object represents a container of sorts (Clark, 1973). Hodun's methodology attempts to equalize this strong action bias with other manipulative actions; her reinforced search task involved a hide and seek game in which children were provided prepositional "clues" that led to the location of a concealed piece of candy. Children were instructed, for example, to look *"under the desk"* for the candy. If the child responded appropriately to the instruction, he was credited with correct comprehension of that preposition; otherwise his systematic search in other spatial locations was recorded until he finally seized the hidden reward. Stimulus objects such as the toy desk were chosen so that they permitted several different spatial prepositions to be equally represented during the search task. In this way, response alternatives for six different prepositions *(in, on, under, front, behind, side)* were equiprobable and minimized the very young child's overriding object or action preferences.

An informal task of this type would be quite easy to construct and administer to the language disabled child and would provide a better estimate of his actual comprehension of spatial terms in the language since object and action biases are characteristically frequent in this clinical population.

In 1958, Jean Berko devised a unique informal assessment tool for examining children's ability to apply morphological rules to novel and unfamiliar stimulus sentences. Berko utilized nonsense stimuli and a sentence completion format that has since been modified for formal assessment purposes, e.g. the Grammatic Closure subtest of the Illinois Test of Psycholinguistic Abilities; Kirk, McCarthy, and Kirk, 1968. In the close technique, two stimuli (pictures or auditory) are presented to the child; the first stimulus is verbally identified by the examiner, e.g. "This is a *wug.*" The second stimulus represents something grammatically different from the first and requires verbal completion by the child, e.g. "These are two _____." Response: *"wugs."* Hence, this task assesses the child's ability to recall and produce various morphological markers that will grammatically conform to and complete the partial sentence.

Language delayed children often manifest a number of specific morphological errors in their conversational speech, e.g. "My feetses hurt," "I wented to the store yesterday," which parallel many of the early morphological deviations in the normal child's speech. An eight-year-old, language delayed child who deletes or inappropriately uses morphological markers such as the possessive [–s] [–z], plural [–s] [–z], [az], or comparative forms of adjectives [–er] in his speech may lack appropriate rule-use of these markers in comprehension. How do we go about resolving this tentative hypothesis? If we already have evidence from the child's spontaneous speech and from his performance on the Grammatic Closure subtest (ITPA) that expressive deficits in the *encoding* of these elements exist, then we should select a test such as Carrow's TALC to further assess the child's ability to *decode* morphological markers and their rule-combinations in the language. In this way we will know whether the child has failed altogether in generating an appropriate set of morphological rules or, alternately, has access to a correct set of rules in comprehension that he has failed to encode.

Thus far in this discussion we have focussed on several measures of language comprehension, realizing that assessment techniques for probing this behaviorally covert modality are yet to be satisfactorily developed. Production abilities in the child are behaviorally more observable and therefore, more amenable to study. Assessment procedures for this language modality have been characteristically divided into two response modes: *elicited imitation* and *spontaneous production*. Menyuk (1963) popularized assessment techniques for the first mode when she discovered that children reproduce modelled sentences that exceed their auditory memory span relative to what they know about grammar. Hence, children seem to practice selectivity in imitating long sentences by preserving grammatical forms with which they are familiar and deleting other structures for which they have not yet induced a set of linguistic rules.

A great deal of psycholinguistic research has documented the "telegraphic" character of the young child's elicited imitations: words and morphemes are selectively omitted from a modelled sentence, making the child's reproductions a grammatically incomplete yet abbreviated version of the original sentence (Miller and Ervin, 1964; Brown and Fraser, 1963; Bloom, 1970). Nevertheless, the child's cognitive and linguistic abilities in handling grammatically complex sentences also underlie length constraints on his imitative utterances. Normal children can repeat model sentences that typically exceed their spontaneous sentence-length if syntactical relationships are not overly difficult but have problems with short complex sentences, such as "Mozart who cried came to my party" (Slobin and Welsh, 1973).

There are numerous other variables known to influence what and how children imitate, including stress factors, word position in the model sentence, semantic cohesiveness, and so forth. These variables will not be discussed, but the clinician is alerted to consider them carefully whenever interpretations of the child's imitative performance are necessary.

Carrow (1974) has constructed an Elicited Inventory of Language (ELI) that formally assesses the child's imitation of several basic sentence construction types; the child repeats fifty-seven sentences that vary in length from two to ten words and that increase in the number of semantic relations and grammatical morphemes. Thus, the child's auditory memory for handling more elements in a sentence and his ability to process increasingly more complex linguistic structures is evaluated by the ELI. All imitative responses are recorded on audio tape and transcribed for later analysis. ELI scoring instructions are quite complex and cannot be practically explained in the text here. However, they do classify the child's incorrect imitations in terms of error type, e.g. addition, substitution, omission, transposition, and reversal errors, and according to the grammatical class each word in the sentence represents. In this way, the child's error profile identifies particular grammatical categories that pose greater difficulty for him.

In addition to being sensitive to various types of grammatical errors reflected in the child's imitative speech, the *ELI* is particularly useful in identifying the nature of children's predicate formation and/or conjugation errors. The ELI has an extensive scoring section devoted to classification of verb errors by *type,* e.g. modal, auxillary, copula, main verb, etc., as well by tense, person, and number aspects of the verb.

One of the drawbacks to the ELI, however, is the disproportionate number of words that represent each of eight different grammatical categories in this test. This shortcoming, in addition to the nonuniform natural frequencies of these word classes appearing in English, should discourage any cross-comparison of percentages of performance on each grammatical category on this test. Sampling problems of this nature arise even in those situations evoking spontaneous speech in the child, so caution is advised whenever clinicians must make interpretations about a child's productive control of various grammatical constituents in the language.

Spontaneous production, as a second type of expressive speech modality, avoids many of the pitfalls introduced by elicited imitation measures. Bloom (1974) has detailed many of these disadvantages and criticizes the validity of elicited imitation in representing children's natural production abilities since imitation procedures impose unrealistic and contextually empty speaking conditions on the child. Consequently, elicited imitation as well as most comprehension measures tell us only what a child can do under *task instruction* rather than what he will do spontaneously with language.

The most viable procedure for assessing a child's natural inclinations for language is sampling his spontaneous speech. Dale (1976) and Lee (1974) have specified a procedural protocol for collecting a language sample from normal and linguistically deviant children, so these techniques will not be detailed in this chapter. Most beginning clinicians lack considerable experience in *analyzing* a language sample, and thus neglect to make this their most useful assessment tool. Fortunately, psycholinguists have done an admirable job in describing children's speech and have constructed some classificatory systems that greatly simplify the task of language analysis. Brown (1973) refined methods for computing the average length of a child's utterances described previously in this chapter as mean length of utterance (MLU). Dale (1976) has summarized the procedures and steps for computing MLU and for assigning children according to Brown's (1973) five stages of linguistic development. Hence, clinicians can roughly determine whether a child's spontaneous language is stage-appropriate or delayed relative to the approximate number of morphemes that appear in his conversational speech.

In addition to measures of verbal output such as MLU, Brown has longitudinally traced the developmental orders of emergence of various grammatical morphemes such as the plural, the present progressive [–ing], past tense, *in* and *on,* and so forth. Although orders were not altogether invariant in the normal children Brown studied, they do provide a basic guideline for determining whether the language disabled child is acquiring expected grammatical structures at a slower than normal rate or whether his grammar is qualitatively deviant and, therefore, *disordered* in some way.

Analysis of syntactic elements and constructions evidenced in the child's speech is not overwhelmingly difficult and has been accomplished in several ways. Brown (1973) and Johnston and Schery (1976) propose one method that is quite successful: determining children's productive use of different syntactic structures (including grammatical morphemes) in communicative contexts that require them. In other words, we compute the percentages of occurrence for a single grammatical element (such as the present progressive [–ing] on verbs) in *obligatory contexts* rather than merely tabulating their absolute frequency in the child's speech. Initially, a list of all utterances in which the present progressive was deleted and used appropriately should be compiled[1]; this list thus represents all obligatory contexts represented in the language sample. Percentages of correct use can then be computed by dividing the *total* number of speech contexts (from above) into the number of contexts in which [–ing] was used appropriately and multiplying this figure by 100.

Johnston and Schery point out that measures of percentage occurrence in obligatory contexts are a valuable assessment device, which can also be used on a longitudinal basis to register

[1]The utterance "He is combing his hair" represents appropriate use of [–ing] in one obligatory context. The utterance "He is walking and run to the store" represents appropriate use of and deletion of [–ing] in *two* obligatory contexts.

any developmental changes in the child's speech.

Brown (1973) and several others have also advanced ways of analyzing children's early utterances in terms of the semantic relationships they express. Frequency measures are perhaps the more common way of representing semantic functions that appear in the child's speech. Like syntactical structures, semantic relationships are known to emerge in a particular developmental sequence; naming functions (nomination) for example are quite prominent in the one– and two-word utterances of young children as are words such as *more, another, again* that all signal the semantic function of *recurrence*.

Hence, semantic relationships reveal not only a child's knowledge of structural relationships in the language, for example that nouns preceding verbs in active declarative sentences identify either the *agent* or *person affected* by the action, but also the child's intended meanings. In contrast, syntactic analysis cannot supply information about communicative intent; it only identifies the grammatical surface structure of a child's utterance. Thus, children's noun-noun combinations can be represented only one way from a syntactic perspective, but they have several possible semantic realizations, e.g. in *possessive* relationships ("doggie dinner" = that's the doggie's dinner), or alternatively in *locative* relationships ("sweater chair" = the sweater is on the chair), or in *agent-object* relationship ("Mommy sock" = Mommy is putting on the sock).

Clinicians can augment the child's communicative competence by assessing and training early-emerging semantic functions in concert with their corresponding syntactical structures in the language.

Although this chapter will not detail techniques for semantic analysis, clinicians are urged to become familiar with them as they appear elsewhere in print (Brown, 1973; Bowerman, 1973; Miller and Yoder, 1974).

Other language-sample-analysis measures used widely by many speech clinicians are those developed by Lee (1974) and her colleagues (1971, 1975). Developmental Sentence Type (DST) analysis was developed for syntactically classifying children's pre-sentence utterances, while Developmental Sentence Scoring (DSS) outlines a developmental sequence of eight grammatical categories for classifying children's grammatically complete sentences. DSS analysis analyzes fifty of the child's spontaneous utterances and assigns a weighted score for each grammatical structure appearing in the sample; higher scores represent structures that appear later in the developmental sequence. Overall DST and DSS scores can then be compared against normative data (Lee, 1974) to determine the child's percentile level of performance and to assess relative amounts of language delay in chronological months. This information permits a prescriptive remedial package to be developed for the child based on the nature and extent of his grammatical deficits (Ruder and Weber-Olsen, in press).

Evaluating Related Aspects of Language Development
Pragmatic Functions

More recently, child language research has directed its efforts to more effectively studying the functional use of language in social contexts and in the child's natural environments. Sociolinguistics is one branch of linguistics that has pioneered methods for assessing the *pragmatic* functions of language, which define how language comes to be used in socially manipulable ways by children. Rules of discourse, politeness rules, context, co-occurring gestures, shared knowledge between speaker and listener, speaker intentions, and other conversational constraints are all pragmatic features, for example, that the child must learn from the social and communicative situations to which he is exposed. In this respect, pragmatic theory acknowledges that language accomplishes socially recognized communicative functions in addition to directly conveying messages or propositional material.

Application of pragmatic theory to clinical assessment and intervention programming of the language disabled is a relatively recent endeavor (cf. Snyder, 1975; Waryas and Stremel-Campbell, in press). Muma (1975) has developed a communication model that addresses the need for teaching the communicative functions as well as structural aspects of language. Various interpersonal communicative tasks devised by Glucksberg, Krauss, and Weisberg (1966) and Longhurst (1972) make the practical assessment of these communicative skills in children a reality. The nature of these tasks involves two individuals assigned to either speaker or listener roles who face each other and attempt to communicate across a visual barrier. The speaker's communicative effectiveness is determined relative to his listener's accuracy in interpreting his message. The message might be realized in a number of ways: for example, by requiring the speaker to describe certain target stimuli contained in an array of stimuli so that the listener will be able to select it from an identical array. Communicative exchanges can be assessed relative to the linguistic sophistication of speaker and listener by increasing the complexity of the stimuli or introducing unfamiliar listeners. Visual barriers can be varied in size to evoke additional communicative cues, e.g. gestures and facial feedback, between speaker and listener (Longhurst and Reichle, 1975). Speaker-listener roles can be exchanged and topic/comment cues introduced to assess production and comprehension of the pragmatic functions of language.

Structured communicative episodes of this type are easily-constructed; if informal tasks for speaker-listener exchanges are appropriately constructed by the clinician, they will prove to be an invaluable assessment tool for evaluating the child's overall communicative competence.

Cognition

Considerable research in child language acquisition has focussed on the child's early prelinguistic and cognitive development. Theoretical assumptions are that these skills serve as prerequisites for the acquisition of early linguistic structures (Slobin, 1970; Sinclair, 1971). If language functions primarily as a code of the child's cognitive knowledge, evaluation of cognitive skills should be a major consideration for language assessment purposes. Nevertheless, it is extremely difficult to devise tasks for assessing the child's cognitive achievements that are also *language independent*. Piaget has pioneered many of the assessment techniques for evaluating cognitive stages of growth in the child, although many of his procedures, such as conservation of mass, volume, and weight tasks, require explicit verbal exchanges between examiner and child. Uzgiris and Hunt (1975) have developed several scales for assessing cognitive functions in infants, which avoid reliance on verbal response channels. Many of their tasks are patterned after sensorimotor skills described by Piaget's work.

Although cognitive achievements are difficult to quantify in the child, clinicians have relied for a great number of years on informal tasks that evaluate children's ability to match colors, objects, sizes, and other nonverbal skills. These can be useful clinical tools for the difficult to test child or for language disabled children with severe to profound intellectual deficits as well. Waryas and Stremel-Campbell (in press) have adapted an assessment battery that includes a comprehensive behavioral checklist and general and specific language tests that evaluate aspects of pre-linguistic communication as well as receptive and expressive skills. Similarly, Muma in his 1978 manuscript, has constructed an assessment paradigm that comprehensively examines cognitive, linguistic, and communicative systems in the child. Muma's procedures provide for the independent assessment of cognitive abilities across several intersecting domains. All cognitive tasks are nonverbal and evaluate, for example, whether a child's major processing mode is oriented towards *perceptual* attributes (iconic processing) vs. *functional* attributes of experience (symbolic processing). Various discrimination tasks determine if children's performance is strongly influenced by perceptually salient cues such as color, size, shape, or position. Other task areas include cognitive distancing skills, primacy-recency functions for memory, and rule– vs. non–rule-governed learning.

Intellectual, perceptual-motor, and hearing assessments all equally contribute to the total clinical picture of the language handicapped child; though they cannot be thoroughly considered here, these topics should not be overlooked in the language assessment process. Nevertheless, it is the bias of this writer that comprehensive and reliable assessments of these developmental abilities in the child require the expertise of professionals trained in these clinical areas. The language clinician should become familiar with clinical tools and methods used by various professional disciplines, for example, in intelligence testing, medical or audiological evaluations, to improve understanding of other parameters of the child's total development and to improve liaisons with professionals whose multidisciplinary efforts can augment habilitation for the language delayed.

Summary

This chapter began by providing an evaluative framework that delineated the *when* and *how* of language assessment. An ongoing means of evaluation that systematically sought the resolution of one or several clinical hypotheses was endorsed as the most advisable timetable and strategy for conducting language evaluations.

For several compelling reasons, a developmental approach to the assessment of language skills in children was adopted for discussion. Various language skills were classified under four basic parameters of linguistic development, including phonological, morphological, syntactical, and semantic developmental skills. Various formal and informal language measures were found to be sensitive to deviations in any one of these four areas of linguistic achievement and, therefore, were recommended for assessment purposes in the basis of how well they helped clarify the nature of the child's language disability.

The advantages and disadvantages of formal and informal evaluation instruments were discussed with emphasis on the need for incorporating both into the clinical assessment of language. Modalities of comprehension and production were comprehensively reviewed next; several formal and informal tests were described and recommended for identifying particular linguistic deficits in the language delayed and disordered child. More recent interests in evaluating the child's knowledge and use of the *communicative* (pragmatic) functions of language was considered in light of the growing need for teaching language in more socially relevant contexts to the language handicapped. Finally, a very brief discussion about cognitive development and its relationship to linguistic development was undertaken, and a few more recent assessment tools that have been used for evaluating these developmental skills in the child were discussed.

Since assessment approaches will vary more dramatically as a function of the individual child rather than the type of language disorder he displays, a single language assessment paradigm was not endorsed in this chapter. However, careful systematic pursuit of the theoretical and clinical issues that reflect on child language development will prepare the beginning clinician for his/

her first assessment experience and will ultimately benefit professional competence.

References

Ammons, R.B. and Ammons, H.S.: Full-Range Picture Vocabulary Test. Missoula, Mont.: Psychological Test Specialists, 1977.

Berko, J.: The child's learning of English morphology. *Word, 14,* 150-177, 1958.

Bloom, L.: *Language Development: Form and Function in Emerging Grammars.* Cambridge, Mass.: MIT Press, 1970.

Bloom, L.: Talking, understanding, and thinking. In R.L. Schiefelbusch and L.L.Lloyd (Eds.): *Language Perspectives—Acquisition, Retardation and Intervention.* Baltimore, Md.: University Park Press, 1974.

Bloom, L., Lightbown, P., and Hood, L.: Structure and variation in child language. *Monogr Soc Res Child Dev, 40,* 1975.

Bowerman, M.: *Early Syntactic Development: A Cross-Linguistic Study with Special Reference to Finnish.* London: Cambridge University Press, 1973.

Bowerman, M.: Commentary to L. Bloom, P. Lightbown, and L. Hood; Structure and variation in child language. *Monogr Soc Res Child Dev, 40(2),* 1975.

Braine, M.D.S.: The ontogeny of English phrase structure: The first phase. *Language, 39(1),* 1-14, 1963.

Braine, M.D.S.: Children's first word combinations. *Monogr Soc Res Child Dev, 41,* 1-104, 1976.

Bricker, W.A. and Bricker, D.D.: An early language training strategy. In R.L. Schiefelbusch and L.L.Lloyd (Ed.): *Language Perspectives—Acquisition, Retardation and Intervention.* Baltimore, Md.: University Park Press, 1974.

Bricker, D., Ruder, K., and Vincent-Smith, L.: An intervention strategy for language deficient children. In R.L. Schiefelbusch and N. Haring (Eds.): *Teaching Special Children.* New York: McGraw-Hill, 1976.

Brown, R., *A First Language.* Cambridge, Mass.: Harvard University Press, 1973.

Brown, R. and Bellugi, U.: Three processes in the child's acquisition of syntax. *Harvard Educ Rev, 34,* 133-151, 1964.

Brown, R., Cazden, C., and Bellugi-Klima, U.: The child's grammar from I to III. In J.P. Hill (Ed.): *Minnesota Symposia on Child Development.* Minneapolis, Minn.: University of Minnesota Press, *2,* 28-73, 1968.

Carrier, J.K.: Application of functional analysis and a nonspeech response mode to teaching language. In L.V. McReynolds (Ed.): Developing systematic procedures for training children's language. *ASHA Monographs, 18,* 47-95, 1974.

Carrier, J.K.: Application of a nonspeech language system with the severely language handicapped. In L.L. Lloyd (Ed.): *Communication Assessment and Intervention Strategies.* Baltimore, Md.: University Park Press, 1976.

Carrow, E.: Test for Auditory Comprehension of Language. Austin, Tex.: Learning Concepts, 1973.

Carrow, E.: Elicited Language Inventory. Austin, Tex.: Learning Concepts, 1974.

Chapman, R.S. and Miller, J.F.: Word order in early two and three-word utterances: Does production precede comprehension? *J Speech Hear Res, 18,* 355-371, 1975.

Chomsky, N.: *Aspects on the theory of syntax.* Cambridge, Mass.: MIT Press, 1965.

Clark, E.V.: Nonlinguistic strategies and the acquisition of word meaning. *Cognition, 2,* 161-182, 1973.

Dale, P.A.: *Language Development: Structure and Form,* 2nd ed. New York: Holt, Rinehart and Winston, 1976.

De Villiers, J.G. and De Villiers, P.A.: A cross-sectional study of the acquisition of grammatical morphemes in child speech. *J Psycholing Res, 2,* 267-278, 1973.

Dunn, L.M. Peabody Picture Vocabulary Test. Circle Pines, Minn.: American Guidance Service, 1959.

Emerick, L. and Hatten, J.T.: *Diagnosis and Evaluation in Speech Pathology.* Englewood Cliffs, N.J.: Prentice-Hall, 1974.

Foster, R., Giddan, J.J., and Stark, J.: *Assessment of Children's Language Comprehension: A Critical Elements Index.* Palo Alto, Calif.: Consulting Psych Press, 1973.

Fraser, C., Bellugi, U., and Brown, R.: Control of grammar in imitation, comprehension and production. *J Verb Learning Verb Behav, 2,* 121-135, 1963.

Glucksberg, S., Krauss, R.M., and Weisberg, R.: Referential communication in nursery school children. *J Exp Psych, 3,* 333-342, 1966.

Goldman, R. and Fristoe, M.: The Goldman Fristoe Test of Articulation. Circle Pines, Minn.: American Guidance Service, 1969.

Graham, L.W.: Language programming and intervention. In L.L. Lloyd (Eds.): *Communication Assessment and Intervention Strategies.* Baltimore, Md.: University Park Press, 1976.

Gray, B.B. and Ryan, B.P.: *A Language Program for the Nonlanguage Child.* Champaign, Ill.: Research Press, 1973.

Guess, D., Sailor, W., and Baer, D.M.: To teach language to retarded children. In R.L. Schiefelbusch and L.L. Lloyd (Eds.): *Language Perspectives—Acquisition, Retardation and Intervention.* Baltimore, Md.: University Park Press, 1974.

Hodun, A.: *Comprehension and the Development of Spatial and Temporal*

Sequence Terms. Unpublished Dissertation, University of Wisconsin, 1975.

Ingram, D.: The relationship between comprehension and production. In R.L. Schiefelbusch and L.L. Lloyd (Eds.): *Language Perspectives—Acquisition, Retardation and Intervention.* Baltimore, Md.: University Park Press, 1974.

Johnston, J.R. and Schery, T.K.: The use of grammatical morphemes by children with communication disorders. In D.M. Morehead and A.E. Morehead (Eds.): *Normal and Deficient Child Language.* Baltimore, Md.: University Park Press, 1976.

Keeney, T. and Wolfe, J.: The acquisition of agreement in English. *J Verb Learning Verb Behav, 11,* 698-705, 1972.

Kirk, S.A., McCarthy, J.J., and Kirk, W.D.: *Illinois Test of Psycholinguistic Abilities* (revised ed.). Urbana, Ill.: University of Illinois Press, 1968.

Lackner, J.R.: A developmental study of language behavior in retarded children. *Neuropsych, 6,* 301-320, 1968.

Lee, L.L., Northwestern Syntax Screening Test. Evanston, Ill.: Northwestern University Press, 1969.

Lee, L.L.: *Developmental Sentence Analysis: A Grammatical Assessment Procedure for Speech and Language Clinicians.* Evanston, Ill.: Northwestern University Press, 1974.

Lee, L.L. and Canter, S.M.: Developmental sentence scoring: A clinical procedure for estimating syntactic development in children's spontaneous speech. *J Speech Hear Dis, 36,* 315-340, 1971.

Lee, L.L., Koenigsknecht, R.A., and Mulhern, S.T.: *Interactive Language Development Teaching: The Clinical Presentation of Grammatical Structure.* Evanston, Ill.: Northwestern University Press, 1975.

Longhurst, T.M.: Assessing and increasing descriptive communicative skills in retarded children. *Ment Retard, 10,* 42-45, 1972.

Longhurst, T.M. and Reichle, J.E.: The applied communication game: A comment on Muma's "communication game: Dump and play." *J Speech Hear Dis, 40,* 315-319, 1975.

MacLeish, A.: *A Glossary of Grammar and Linguistics.* New York: Grosset and Dunlap, 1971.

McNeill, D.: Developmental psycholinguistics. In F. Smith and G.A. Miller (Eds.): *The Genesis of Language.* Cambridge, Mass.: MIT Press, 1966.

McNeill, D.: *The Acquisition of Language: The Study of Developmental Psycholinguistics.* New York: Harper and Row, 1970.

Menyuk, P.: A preliminary evaluation of grammatical capacity in children. *J Verb Learning Verb Behav, 2,* 429-439, 1963.

Menyuk, P. and Looney, P.L.: Relationships among components of the grammar in language disorders. *J Speech Hear Res, 15,* 395-406, 1972.

Miller, J.F. and Yoder, D.E.: An ontogen language teaching strategy for retarded children. In R.L. Schiefelbusch and L.L. Lloyd (Eds.): *Language Perspectives—Acquisition, Retardation and Intervention.* Baltimore, Md.: University Park Press, 1974.

Miller, W.R. and Ervin, S.M.: The development of grammar in child language. In U. Bellugi and R. Brown (Eds.): The Acquisition of Language. *Monogr Soc Res Child Dev, 29,* 9-33, 1964.

Morehead, D.M. and Ingram, D.: The development of base syntax in normal and linguistically deviant children. *J Speech Hear Res, 16,* 330-352, 1973.

Muma, J.R.: *Language Handbook: Concepts, Assessment, Intervention.* Englewood Cliffs, Prentice-Hall, 1978.

Muma, J.R.: The communication game: Dump and Play. *J Speech Hear Dis, 40,* 296-309, 1975.

Nelson, K.: Structure and strategy in learning to talk. *Monogr Soc Res Child, 149,* 1973.

Premack, D.: Language in chimpanzee? *Science, 172,* 808-822, 1971.

Prutting, C.A., Gallagher, T.M. and Mulac, A.: The expressive portion of the NSST compared to a spontaneous language sample. *J Speech Hear Dis, 40,* 40-48, 1975.

Ratusnik, D.L. and Koenigsknecht, R.A.: Internal consistency of the NSST. *J Speech Hear Dis, 40,* 59-68, 1975.

Ruder, K.F. and Weber-Olsen, M.: Psycholinguistic based language training: Application to language delay and mental retardation. To appear in K.F. Ruder and M.D. Smith (Eds.): *Applied Psycholinguistics,* in press.

Rumbaugh, D. (Ed.): *Language Learning in the Chimpanzee.* New York: Academic Press, 1977.

Schultz, M.C.: The bases of speech pathology and audiology: evaluation as the resolution of uncertainty. *J Speech Hear Dis, 38,* 147-155, 1973.

Schultz, M.C. and Carpenter, M.A.: The bases of speech pathology and audiology: What are appropriate models? *J Speech Hear Dis, 38,* 395-404, 1974.

Shriner, T.H., Holloway, M.S., and Daniloff, R.G.: The relationship between articulatory deficits and syntax in speech defective children. *J Speech Hear Res, 12,* 319-325, 1969.

Sinclair-deZwart, H.: Sensorimotor action patterns as a condition for the acquisition of syntax. In R. Huxley and E. Ingram (Eds.): *Language Aquisition: Models and Methods.* New York: Academic Press, 1971.

Slobin, D.I.: Cognitive prerequisites for the development of grammar. Reprinted from W.O. Dingwall (Ed.): *A Survey of Linguistic Science.* College Park: University of Maryland Linguistics Program, 1970.

Slobin, D.I. and Welsh, C.A.: Elicited imitation as a research tool in developmental psycholinguistics. In C.A. Ferguson and D.I. Slobin (Eds.):

Studies of Child Language Development. New York: Holt, Rinehart and Winston, 1973.

Snyder, L.: *Pragmatics in Langauge Disabled Children: Their Prelinguistic and Early Verbal Performatives and Presuppositions.* Unpublished dissertation, University of Colorado, 1975.

Stremel, K. and Waryas, C.: A behavioral-psycholinguistic approach to language training. In L.V. McReynolds (Ed.): Developing systematic procedures for training children's language. *ASHA Monogr, 18,* 1974.

Templin, M.C.: The study of articulation and language development during the early school years. In F. Smith and G.A. Miller (Eds.): *The Genesis of Language: A Psycholinguistic Approach.* Cambridge, Mass.: MIT Press, 1966.

Templin, M. and Darley, F.: The Templin-Darley Test of Articulation. Iowa City, Bureau of Educational Research and Service, University of Iowa Press, 1969.

Uzgiris, I. and Hunt, J. McV.: *Assessment in Infancy: Ordinal Scales of Psychological Development.* Urban, Univ of Illinois Press; 1975.

Waryas, C.A. and Ruder, K.F.: On the limitations of language compre, hension procedures and an alternative. *J Speech Hear Dis, 39,* 44-52, 1974.

Waryas, C.A. and Stremel-Campbell, K.: Grammatical training for the language delayed child. A new perspective. To appear in R.L. Schiefelbusch (Ed.): *The Bases of Language Intervention.* Baltimore, Md.: University Park Press, in press.

Winitz, H.: *Articulatory Acquisition and Behavior.* New York: Appleton-Century-Crofts, 1969.

Chapter 2

TECHNIQUES FOR CHILDREN
WITH DEVIANT LANGUAGE

JULIA R. BOXX

Purpose

L ANGUAGE DISABILITY in children takes a multitude of forms. The term *deviant language* will be used here in its broadest sense to mean language skills that are not at their expected level. It is not the purpose of this chapter to detail the causes or nature of various forms of deviant language. Neither will the issue of "what" to train be discussed, as the needs of each language-deviant child differ, at least to some degree, from those of other language-deviant children. A thorough language assessment as discussed in Chapter 1 should provide information regarding the particular area or areas of language skills, the "what," that are needed.

Rather, this chapter will present a number of techniques that have been found useful in reducing or overcoming a child's deviant language. These techniques should prove helpful to speech pathologists, parents, teachers, and other persons involved with a language-deviant child in establishing adequate language skills. The techniques discussed are not intended to be procedures specific to the remediation of only one parameter of language. They should lend themselves to the remediation of all, or at least several, parameters, whether the disability is semantic, morphologic, syntactic, or some combination thereof.

Criteria for Determining the Value of a Technique

The general purpose of any technique used in a language therapy program is to facilitate the child's use of adequate language skills. A technique should assist the child in his internalizing of a rule or set of rules for a particular language. It is impossible to train every possible word, phrase, and sentence the child will ever need or want to use. Thus, language remediation techniques must isolate and present clear examples of the rules, which the child must identify and learn. In learning this finite set of rules, the child will then be equipped to generate an infinite number of appropriate utterances.

Everyone working with the language-deviant child will have some particular ideas about what makes a technique useful and worthwhile. It would seem, however, that the following criteria might be agreed to by most of those persons in deciding if a technique meets its general purpose. These criteria include that a technique must —

1. be applicable across the training of a number of language forms, i.e. semantic, morphologic, syntactic;
2. be easy for the child to grasp or participate in successfully;
3. afford the child a high rate of successful responses;
4. be easy for the person working with the child to set up and carry out efficiently;
5. effect a positive change in the child's language skills in a short period of time;
6. aid the child in generalizing what is learned to untrained items;
7. enable the child to transfer his new skills to situations outside a structured remedial situation.

While this sounds like a large order for any technique to fill, it does give the instructor some things to think about, and helps to avoid the use of a technique that does little more than "fill up time" with the child. With at least these criteria in mind, the person working with a language-deviant child should be able to evaluate the usefulness of a technique as one possibly to be included in a language remediation program. The techniques discussed in the next section are ones that have been found, through research and clinical programs, to be effective in remediating language disability in young children.

Of course, not all of these techniques would be necessary for any one child, nor would all be directly applicable to every child. Nonetheless, they should provide the instructor some ideas for beginning or enhancing a language remediation program.

Techniques for Language Remediation with Children

Modeling

Cazden (1972) identified modeling as one technique mothers use to enhance communication with their children. Modeling broadens the child's semantic framework. It offers the child more semantic information about a particular situation. It can be used before or after the child makes a comment. The following conversation examples modeling.

> Antecedent: adult begins a conversation with child.
> Mother: "We need to go to the store to buy groceries."
>
> Subsequential: adult comments on child's utterance without correcting or repeating.
> Child: "Us go store now?"
> Mother: "Yes, and we'll buy some candy when we get there.

The mother is offering more information to the child. While her sentence structure is more elaborate, it is not her primary intent to offer the child a more complex sentence, but rather to offer additional meaningful content. This technique is useful clinically in that it gives the child more things to "think about" and thus to comment upon to the listener. Further, the child is presented with different sentence types and structures than those he used, but which are still relevant to his topic area.

This technique has at least two strong points. These are (1) that it draws from what the child says to extend the child's comments and (2) it does not correct or repeat the child's syntactic forms. Thus, it does not require that a child produce a form that he may be unable to do correctly except as rote imitation word by word.

Expansion

This technique is used to reformulate the child's utterance into an adultlike form either semantically or syntactically. Brown (1973) found that mothers expand both the child's semantic and his syntactic forms, but are more concerned with the "truth value" or semantic aspect of what the child says than with the correctness of syntax. The procedure is exampled below.

Grammatical Expansion: Child—Here doggie house.
                        Mother—Here's the doggie's house.

Semantic Expansion: Child—We went to Dallas, Texas.
                        Mother—No, we went to *Houston,*
                        Texas, not Dallas.

As the examples illustrate, the adult has restated, in an adultlike form for the child, what the child said. This technique provides the child greater accuracy, either semantically or grammatically, if not both. In this way, the child becomes more readily understood by the listener. When an utterance is wrong or quite primitive, it becomes more difficult for the listener to grasp the meaning. By expanding the child's utterances to an adultlike level, or at least to a level higher than the child's own, the instructor can show the child how to get his specific message across more effectively. Expansions also help the adult to better understand what the child meant. By expanding the child's utterance, the adult can determine if that was in fact what the child intended to say. The child's response to the expansion may be "No!" indicating something else was meant, or "Uh-huh" indicating agreement.

Expansion was also identified by Cazden (1972) as another way in which mothers verbally interact with their children. In a controlled study, Cazden attempted to determine which technique, modeling or expansion, had the greater effect on language development. In this study, modeling was found to be the more effective of the two. Other research, however, (Feldman and Rodgon, 1970) has shown no differences between the two techniques, and both expansion and modeling are widely used to improve language skills in children even now.

One difficulty that may occur when using expansion is that it may limit the child's meaning at times. This could occur if the child is using a set of words to mean something that they do not mean to the adult or if the child is using words as different parts of speech than they would be used as by the adult. Many researchers (Bloom, 1970; Bowerman, 1976; Clark, 1974; Leonard, 1977) have found that even the young language-normal child does not always use words in the same way adults use those same words. Thus, the child's utterance may not retain its original meaning when reformulated into an adultlike sentence. When the child's general meaning is, however, somewhat obvious, expansion does provide it a more elaborate form and, in many cases, assists the adult in figuring out what the child intended to say.

Forced Wrong Choices

Many times the language-deviant child will use seemingly inappropriate forms such as "him go," "boy play," "girls eats," or "her jumpeded." These forms may have a logical, rule-governed pattern, which is not always apparent to the listener. The forced wrong choice technique identifies that aspect of the sentence, if any, to which the child is attending to gain or to convey information. This technique presents the child with two choices, both of which are wrong. Waryas and Ruder (1974) present an assessment procedure for comprehension using this type of procedure. It can, however, be used effectively as a therapy tool as well. Two examples of this technique follow. A picture of a boy pulling a wagon is shown to the child. Then two sentences are said to the child. These might be, "She pulls the wagon" and "Him pulls the wagon." The first sentence is syntactically correct but semantically incorrect, while the second is syntactically incorrect but semantically correct. The child is to choose the sentence that best describes the picture. If the child chooses the first, he might be relying on the grammaticality to identify the picture. If he chooses the second, he might be relying more on the semantics to identify what is said.

A second example is to present two pictures to the child. The first might be of a dog barking and the other of several dogs barking. A sentence is then said to the child. It would be, "The dog bark" or "The dogs barks." The child is then to point to the picture that he thinks the sentence describes. Neither sentence is correct, but the child's pointing response, assuming it is not random guessing, should offer information as to the process the child uses to derive his choice. In this example, his choice would indicate whether he attends to the noun form or the verb form to identify singular versus plural. With this sort of information, the clinician can then direct the child's attention to the aspect of language structure that is not being focused on while simultaneously capitalizing on the form the child uses. These two, the one the child uses and the one he does not, can then be coupled together to enhance his skill over more than one variable.

Further, the forced wrong choice technique would offer the child some freedom to use the processes he has, as there is no concern about having to get a right answer. Lastly, it enables the instructor to identify what language rule or rules the child does have, to compare these to the rules he should have, and thereby, to better understand the child's approach to language learning. By using what the child already knows, the instructor can more successfully aid the child in establishing and generalizing forms not yet known.

Verbal Imitation

The role of imitation as a means of developing language is a controversial one. Several authors (Carrow, 1974; McNeill, 1970; Menyuk, 1963) contend the child will not imitate those structures that are beyond his own level of linguistic competence. Others feel the child may imitate higher forms than he has competence for provided the sentence to be imitated is within the child's memory span (Slobin and Welsh, 1971). Regardless of its impact on the developmental process of language acquisition, verbal imitation is a widely used technique and has been found to be useful in achieving spontaneous production (Ruder and Hermann, 1973; Ruder et al., 1974).

It is common for the adult, in trying to help the child talk better, to have the child imitate his sounds or words. This technique is exampled below.

Parent: "Say what I say. We go to grandma's house."
Child: "We go grama house."
Parent: "We go TO grandma's house."
Child: "We go GRAMA house."

This brief example illustrates some of the difficulty that can occur when the child is expected to imitate structures that are too far beyond his own level of competence. The important thing to remember when using verbal imitation as technique is to use it only for a particular form or set of forms that are just slightly above the child's own present level of functioning. Second, it should be kept in mind that the sentence to imitate ought not to greatly exceed the child's memory span. If these two factors are ignored, what usually results is the child's approximating syntactically what is said to him, rather than grasping the new form and making use of it himself. This approximating utterance, or type of imitative behavior, is what McNeill (1970) terms "resemblance." He comments that this sort of imitation process does play some role in language development, compared to what he calls "technical" imitation, or the *exact* repetition of a sentence, which may be of little value as a procedure for developing language. Thus, the instructor might want to use both of McNeill's types of imitation procedure, depending upon what he or she is trying to accomplish at a particular point.

Fraser, Bellugi, and Brown (1963) found that young children were better able to verbally imitate sentences than they were able to accurately comprehend or produce those same sentences. From this the researchers concluded that imitation is a perceptual-motor task rather than one requiring any processing of language rules. While Fraser, Bellugi, and Brown's finding does not imply that imitation is the predecessor of comprehension and production, it does suggest that imitation of sentences appears to be an easier task than the other two. If this is the case, the imitation of a particular structure within the context of a sentence the child can produce might at least assist the child in becoming aware of the new structure to be acquired. Additionally, imitation of this new structure within the sentence would provide the child with an example of where and how the new structure relates to other aspects of the sentence, which the child already knows. While it is debatable whether imitation plays a role in the child's acquisition of language rules, it does seem evident that this technique may serve to "atune" the child to parts of a sentence that he is currently not aware of or using.

Echoing

With this technique, the adult echos the child's utterance back to him. The adult may use a *Wh–* word such as *what* or *where* in place of an unintelligible word from the child, or he may echo the child's utterance with a rising intonation as if to question what the child said. The following examples illustrate.

Child: "Me got two (unintelligible) "
Adult: "You got two what?"

     •   •   •

Child: "Billy got a new bike."
Adult: "Billy got a new *bike?*"

This technique need not always require that the child respond with any particular sort of answer, or that he respond at all. It does, however, let the child know that at least some of what he says is understood by an adult. Further, it specifies to the child which part of his comment was not understood, thus enabling the child to focus on particular parts rather than having to reiterate his entire comment. Lastly, echoing aids the adult in making sure he or she did understand what the child said, or in clarifying what was not initially understood.

Binary Choices

Often, the parent or clinician does not understand what the child is trying to say, either because the child is unintelligible or does not make sense with his choice of word combinations. The adult, by using the technique of binary choices, can often establish some limits on the child's possible range of answers and can in this way have a better means of understanding the child's response. The following three examples show how this technique may be used.

Adult: "Do you want milk or juice?"
Child: "ooge" (juice)

· · ·

Adult: "Did daddy come home or go to the store?"
Child: "Store bye-bye"

· · ·

Adult: "For dinner we'll have meatloaf or chicken."
Child: "I wi (like or want) memoh (meatloaf) a di (dinner)"

· · ·

By presenting the child with two or more possible acceptable choices, the adult is narrowing the range of responses he will have to figure out. Additionally, this technique eliminates the frustrating situation in which both the child and the adult find themselves when the child must repeat himself over and over, usually without success, to be understood. Such a situation leads everyone concerned to the conclusion that "whenever talking is involved, it's going to be awful," or worse yet, that "it's not worth the hassle."

By using a binary choice technique, this potential "failure" situation can instead become extremely successful for the child and the adult.

The binary choice technique could also be used effectively to help the child compare and contrast language concepts and to stabilize new language forms. The following example illustrates how this can be done.

The child has been learning the regular past tense verb and the regular present tense verb. The clinician holds up a picture of a boy jumping over a rock.

Clinician: "Which sentence is about this picture, "The boy jumps' or 'The boy jumped'?"
Child: "Boy jumps."
Clinician: "That's right. The boy jumps over the rock."

From this example and those given earlier, it can be seen that the binary choice technique is effective in developing the child's semantic and syntactic skills. One of its major advantages is that is can be used in a wide variety of situations and to develop many areas of language skill.

Nonsense Items

Occasionally, the clinician may question whether the child with deviant language is actually using a rule to generate utterances or whether the child is saying a particular word or phrase that he has rotely memorized. It is generally realized that young children produce some memorized forms. These are evidenced by the child's use of nursery rhymes, counting in sequence, and social expressions such as "you bet," "thanks," "get lost," and "just fine." The use of some memorized forms, in itself, is not a problem. When a child is trying to develop language skills, however, relying on the method or process of memorizing can be severely detrimental in that it limits the child to a finite number of sentences. Also, it reduces the likelihood that the child will be able to communicate effectively in new or different situations where those memorized forms are not appropriate or where other forms are not recognized as similar or identical to those memorized.

One way of avoiding the child's possible memorization of words and phrases is to use nonsense words or syllables that have no prior meaning for the child. In this way, the child is encouraged to attend to and learn the rules that are applicable across both familiar and unfamiliar speaking situations.

Berko (1958) conducted a study using nonsense words to determine if children did use rules to produce language and further to determine at what age certain rules were acquired. An example of Berko's procedure follows.

The child was shown two pictures, one of a nonmeaningful, animal-like form and the other of two of these forms. The examiner said, "This is a wug (pointing to the single-item picture). Now there is another one (pointing to the multiple-item picture). There are two of them. There are two _____." The child was to produce a word to finish the sentence. If the child responded with the plural form "wugs," it could be assumed he had the rule for this regular plural marker, as the child could not have memorized a term he had not heard before or been familiar with. As Berko's study was carried out to identify the order in which inflectional endings are acquired, her procedure was not developed as a clinical technique to remediate language disability. It does, nonetheless, serve as such in that it removes meaningful parts of an utterance if the instructor chooses to use it in this way. The meaningful parts are then replaced with nonsense words to focus the child's attention on a particular rule or concept. This technique can be used to train not only regular plural markers, as in the example given, but also other inflectional endings, such as possessive, present progressive, and past tense. It can also be effective in directing the child's attention to different parts of speech within the sentence, such as nouns, verbs, prepositions, adjectives, or adverbs. This is demonstrated in the following example.

> Teacher: "This wug is bizzing fast. How is the wug bizzing?"
> Child: "Fast."
> Teacher: "That's right. Show me how you biz fast."
> Child makes a fast motion of any sort.
> Teacher: "Good for you. What else can you do fast?"
> Child: demonstrates another action or tells teacher.

In this example, the child is attending to an adverb. The wug could be an oddly cut piece of cardboard and the bizzing action could be the cardboard being moved back and forth rapidly by the teacher. In this example, the noun and verb forms are nonmeaningful to the child. The teacher would use many such examples to establish the concept of adverbs, or words that describe actions, or other descriptive words. Further, the teacher might choose to make the adverb a nonsense word and the other parts of speech real words. This sort of contrasting of real to nonsense should sharpen the child's awareness of how the part of speech works. As the example illustrates, the nonsense words can and in many instances should be used not only in what is said, but also in pictures and objects used and in actions demonstrated. In this way, the child is less likely to mentally pair the nonsense word to an already familiar object or activity, e.g. why call a dog a niz?, an occurrence which could lead to great confusion.

This technique works well as a way to improve both comprehension and production skills. While it is an easy and fun task for the child to deal with, it does take much forethought and planning by the instructor.

Sentence Completions

The sentence completion technique is well known and widely used as a testing procedure. It works very well as a training procedure as well, in that it can provide as much or as little assistance to the child as is needed. It can be used to establish a variety of language skills. The six examples presented demonstrate just some of the ways in which this technique might be used.

Clinician: Showing the child a picture and saying, "The boy is ———."

Child: Looking at picture of a boy skating says, "Skating."

· · ·

Clinician: "The boy threw the ———."
Child: "Ball."

· · ·

Clinician: "This boy is laughing. He did the same thing yesterday. What did he do yesterday?"
Child: "Laughed," or "He laughed," or "Boy laughed."

· · ·

Clinician: "You use a hammer to ———."
Child: "Pound nails," or "Hit nails," or "Build things."

· · ·

Clinician: "The boy ———."
Child: "Is eating his lunch and talking to his friend."

As these examples illustrate, the sentence completion technique may be used to elicit a certain word, inflectional ending, or phrase. As the child advances, this technique enables the clinician to reduce the amount of stimuli needed to elicit a response and can allow for a variety of responses to be acceptable.

A variation of this technique is to have the child begin a sentence with those structures he is learning and allow the clinician to finish the sentence. This encourages the child to initiate language activity, using what he knows. This variation is as follows:

The child is working on plurals and prepositions.
Child: "Boys jump on ———."
Clinician: "The trampoline."

· · ·

Child: "Girls play in _____."
Clinician: "Their sandbox."

Either variation of the technique presents information in a structured way to the child. Another advantage of the sentence completion technique is that it can be used across all levels of language complexity, from the one-word response level through more elaborate or advanced multi-word response levels. Use of an already familiar technique with the child, far from boring him as he advances in language skills, offers him the opportunity to focus totally on the new forms without having to learn a new procedure as well.

Error Identification

DeVilliers and DeVilliers (1972) found that young children developing language normally were able to identify, with at least some degree of accuracy, semantic and syntactic errors in sentences presented to them. Only the older children in their study, however, were able to make appropriate corrections of syntax. Both younger and older children were able to make semantic corrections in most instances. These findings suggest that, while a child may not always be able to correct or accurately form a sentence, he may have some knowledge of what makes the sentence acceptable or unacceptable.

If a language impaired child is to establish appropriate forms or modify inappropriate ones, he would be better able to do this if he had some initial notion of whether what he hears is correct or appropriate. The error identification technique enables the child to sort out a sentence himself and to demonstrate something of the processes he uses to determine if the sentence is acceptable. The examples below suggest some ways this technique may be used.

Teacher: "Is this sentence right? 'Him goed the to store'."
Child: "No."
Teacher: "Good for you. Now you try to make it right."
Child: "Him went to the store."

•   •   •

Teacher: "Is this sentence right? 'The cookie ate the boy'."
Child: "No, cause a cookie can't do that. A boy eat a cookie!"

• • •

Teacher: "Is this sentence OK?   The bed pushed a boy."
Child: "No, that silly! A boy pusheded a bed!"

These examples show how a child may be able to recognize a sentence as wrong. Even though his attempts at correction may not be totally adequate, they do tell the teacher something of what the child knows about how the language works. These error identifications and corrections of semantics, syntax, or both indicate also what the child does not yet know or has learned inappropriately.

The error identification technique is particularly useful as a means of stabilizing a new language behavior that has just been acquired. Once the child knows what a language form is and when to use it, this technique provides the child a means of sharpening his knowledge of how the newly acquired form works and when not to use it as well. For example, the teacher might use the new form in an inappropriate context as well as in an appropriate one. The child would be expected to identify where the form was used correctly and incorrectly, thus improving his own knowledge of the rule.

Questions

It is accepted that one of our most effective ways of getting a response from someone is to pose a question. There are three types of questions, all of which are useful as techniques. These are the question that requires a yes-no response, one that requires a naming response as in "What is that?", and the one that requires an open-ended response. The first two types of questions are self-explanatory. The third type will be discussed here.

Lee (1974) points out that, in eliciting a language sample from the child, the open-ended question tends to be the most effective type, as it requires more language usage than either the yes-no question or the question requiring a one-word naming response. The open-ended question technique is exampled here.

Mother: "How did you brush your teeth?"
Child: "With a brush and the paste."

• • •

Mother: "What did you do with the tissue?"

Child: "Blow my nose."
Mother: "Why did you get more tissues?"
Child: "I got lot a runny nose."

The open-ended question allows the child several possible answers, whereas the yes-no or naming type of question requires that the child respond with one specific word if he is to be correct. Certainly these two latter question types can be useful, particularly when the child is extremely limited in expressive language skills. But further, they can, in many instances, be restrictive for the child. Even should the correct one-word response be given to a yes-no question, it may still be necessary to extend further to be sure the child's response was not correct merely by chance guessing alone. Not only does the open-ended question give the child the opportunity of responding with a variety of appropriate answers, but further, it makes for a higher likelihood of successful responses.

Semantic Cueing

This technique is useful when the child has responded inappropriately or is at a loss to respond at all (Wiig and Semel, 1976). Semantic cueing provides the child with related information that may elicit the target response. The following example demonstrates how this technique works.

Clinician: "What is this?"
Child: "I don't know."
Clinician: "It's not a big grown-up dog. It's a baby dog. What else do we call baby dogs?"
Child: "Oh, a puppy. It's a puppy!"

As this example shows, the child can be aided by semantic cues to retrieve a label that he may not be able to spontaneously recall. This technique assumes the child has some knowledge of the form expected, but is unable to retrieve or use it readily. Further, this technique can be used to establish new words or concepts, in that the new information can be paired through cues to what the child already knows. Lastly, semantic cueing encourages the child to do some processing to derive a response rather than merely telling him the specific response required.

Sentence Rearrangement

If the child has the ability to use one– or two-word utterances to label persons, things, and activities, this technique can facilitate his ability to organize his words into a meaningful comment. The first example shows how this technique can elicit an appropriate response, and the second shows how it can be used to overcome the child's error.

Clinician: Showing the child a picture of a boy petting a dog, says, "Here are some words that go with this picture. You put them together in the right way to tell me about the picture. *Boy, dog, petting.*"

Child: "Boy pet dog."

•   •   •

Clinician: Same context as example one.

Child: "Boy dog pet."

Clinician: "No, dog isn't something the boy *does*. What does the boy do to the dog?"

Child: "Pet dog. Him pet puppy."

Employing this technique, the clinician can make use of words the child already has and can provide a meaningful picture or "acting out" scene with toys to help the child see the order and relationship of these words in a sentence.

Bowerman (1976) comments that a "language training program must aim not only at encouraging children to link linguistic forms and devices with categories of experience but also at helping them to improve on their initial guesses about these categories when they are incorrect." One advantage of this technique is that it offers a way of doing this. It provides the words from which the child can create his own sentence by analyzing relationships between these words and categories of experiences. This technique can be used to develop many levels of language skill. It is applicable to the development of early two– and three-word utterances, more complex sentences incorporating articles, prepositions, the auxiliary, and even to sentences containing embedded or subordinate clauses.

Categorizing

This technique is useful in showing the child the relationships between words. Like sentence rearrangment, it is used to help the child see the way words go together to make sense. This technique is based on the notion that a child uses language forms in a way that relates to what he knows conceptually to be the case. The child's earliest attempts to use language take a semantic framework rather than a syntactic one. For example, the child initially will identify animate forms as the "doer" in a sentence and inanimate forms as the "receiver" of an action. Thus, the sentence "The boy eats the cookie" is meaningful whereas "The cookie eats the boy" is not. The meaningfulness is not derived from the relationship of the subject and the object, but rather from the relationship between the doer and the receiver of the action, in short the agent and the object.

The categorizing technique is used to facilitate the child's ability to identify and use words in ways which make sense conceptually. By categorizing words as "doers," "receivers," or "actions," for example, the child has a better chance of grasping the meaning of a sentence. For example:

Clinician: "Show me the ones that can *do* things like run or hit or laugh or play."

Child: points to boy, man, and baby.

Clinician: "Good! Now which ones can't do anything like that?"

Child: Points to table, tree, car, and house.

Clinician: "That's right. Now which sentence is silly, 'The boy hits the table' or 'The table hits the boy'?"

Child: "A table no hits. That silly. Boy hit table."

In this example, the child is categorizing words by whether they are animate or inanimate, and on this basis, he is able to determine which sentence make sense and which does not. While this example is a less complex level of sentence production or comprehension, the technique can be used for more complex forms as well. These might include sentences containing direct and indirect objects, active versus passive word order, or sentences that have the subject and verb separated by an embedded clause.

If the child is able to categorize words by their function, he is more likely to comprehend and produce meaningful sentences. This technique focuses the child's attention towards the function of different words and word classes. Thus, it prepares the child to combine words into meaningful relationships even on a structurally complex level of language development.

Demonstrating Actions

As its name implies, this technique involves the physical acting out of what is said. The child and the instructor physically go through the action as it is being discussed. This technique is intended to tie the linguistic form to the event itself in a concrete way. For example, the instructor and the child pound the Play-Doh® as the instructor talks about "pounding," or the instructor says "We're jumping" as the child and instructor do the action. The real physical action paired to the language provides the child a more perceptually salient context than does a picture and involves the child more directly as a participant.

This technique is quite useful with the very young child who may become bored unless physically active and involved in a situation. It also works well for the child whose language skills are at a very early level, which requires a more concrete tie-together of the language structures and the experiences they represent.

Commands

The use of commands or directives can be employed for development of both comprehension and production skills. The command technique can be paired with other techniques, as "demonstrating actions" just discussed. The command technique can also be used effectively with children at all levels of language learning, in that commands can be made very simple or complex. This technique is exampled below.

Clinician: "You stand up."
Child: Stands up.
Clinician: "Put the ball on the table."
Child: Does as requested.
Clinician: "Find the doll with the red dress, yellow hat, and

white shoes" (might be from a group of dolls dressed differently.)

In the above example, the child is expected to comprehend the instruction and then demonstrate his comprehension by accurately doing as told. In this next example, the command technique is used another way.

The child gives the command, as in saying to the clinician, "Go there," "put the doll in the box," or "Get Play-Doh® and make it a ball." This variation on the command technique is powerful, in that it teaches the child that he can have some degree of control over his environment by using language. Further, it allows him the chance to productively use those commands which he was given by the clinician.

Story Telling

The story telling technique can be used in a number of ways to achieve a variety of goals. Byrne and Shervanian (1977) comment that it can help the child to sequence ideas, to retain information, and to use particular words, inflectional endings, and sentence types. It serves as a type of structured conversational speech. The instructor might tell a story and then ask the child questions related to what was said. These questions could require yes-no, naming, or open-ended responses, depending upon the child's level of skill.

Additionally, the child might be expected to make up a story himself using a set of pictures arranged in sequential order. The child might ask questions of the instructor about the story, or tell the story and make up another ending or event for the story. This technique is an effective one for developing both comprehension and production skills, and it can be tailored to the child's level of semantic and syntactic complexity. Story telling is often used with other techniques, such as questions, sentence completion, binary choices, or imitation, as a means of stabilizing new language forms. As a type of structured conversational speech, it aids in the generalization of what has been learned.

Marketed Language Programs

In addition to the techniques outlined, which by no means are considered to be the only ones used, there are a large number of marketed language training programs available. These programs are usually designed to be used by a particular group, such as classroom teachers, the speech and language clinicians, or parents. These programs may deal with one or several of the parameters of language, e.g. the sound system, semantics, morphology, or syntax. As these programs include detailed discussions of how they are to be used, this section will not outline the procedures of each. Rather, five widely used programs of the many available will be listed here. The interested reader will be able to obtain information about the program from the publisher.

Interactive Language Development Teaching
Authors: Laura L. Lee, Roy A. Koenigsknecht, Susan T. Mulhern
Publishers: Northwestern University Press
                    Evanston, Illinois
Year of Publication: 1975
Area of Emphasis: Morphology and Syntax.

The Grammatical Analysis of Language Disability: A Procedure for Assessment and Remediation
Authors: David Crystal, Paul Fletcher, Michael Garmen
Publishers: Edward Arnold (Publishers) Ltd.
                    25 Hill Street
                    London, England
Year of Publication: 1976
Area of Emphasis: Morphology and Syntax.

Distar
Authors: Siegfried Engelmann, Jean Osborn
Publishers: Science Research Associates, Inc.
                    259 East Erie
                    Chicago, Illinois
Year of Publication: 1972
Area of Emphasis: Concepts, Morphology, and Syntax.

Peabody Language Development Kits
Authors: Lloyd Dunn, J.O. Smith, Katherine Horton

Publishers: American Guidance Service
             Circle Pines, Minnesota
Year of Publication: 1965
Area of Emphasis: Semantics, Morphology, and Syntax.

Gray-Ryan Program for the Non-Language Child
Authors: Burl Gray, Bruce Ryan
Publishers: Research Press
             Champaign, Illinois
Year of Publication: 1973
Area of Emphasis: Morphology and Syntax.

These programs and many others similar to them are detailed and comprehensive. However, as a child should not be made to fit a language program, the instructor must decide if the program or parts of it meet the needs of the individual child. The value of such language programs should be considered by the same criteria one uses to determine the value of any clinical technique. If the program meets the instructor's criteria, its use would be appropriate, but if it does not, it should not be used merely because it is available and already organized.

Summary

This chapter has presented techniques for the improvement of language skills in the language-deviant child. It has discussed (1) criteria for determining the value of a technique, (2) a number of clinical techniques that have been found to be helpful in overcoming deviant language and in establishing appropriate language structures, and (3) a brief discussion of marketed language programs with a listing of five such programs currently in wide use.

The techniques discussed are intended to be applicable at many levels of language training. They may be used individually or in conjunction with one another. The same could be said of any technique and the language programs listed. These techniques and their examples are by no means exhaustive of those available. It is presumed the capable adult working with the language-deviant child will certainly find ways to modify, extend, and enhance these techniques even further to help the child achieve the best language skills possible.

References

Berko, J.: The child's learning of English morphology. *Word, 14,* 150-177, 1958.

Bloom, L.: *Language Development: Form and Function in Emerging Grammars.* Cambridge, Mass.: MIT Press, 1970.

Bowerman, M.: Semantic factors in the acquisition of rules for word use and sentence construction. In D.M. Morehead and A.E. Morehead (Eds.): *Normal and Deficient Child Language.* Baltimore, Md.: University Park Press, 1976.

Brown, R.: *A First Language: The Early Stages.* Cambridge, Mass.: Harvard University Press, 1973.

Byrne, M.C. and Shervanian, C.C.: *Introduction to Communication Disorders.* New York, N.Y.: Harper and Row Publishers, 1977.

Carrow, E.: *Carrow Elicited Language Inventory.* Austin, Tex.: Learning Concepts, 1974.

Cazden, D.: *Child Language and Education.* New York, N.Y.: Holt, Rinehart and Winston, 1972.

Clark, E.: Some aspects of the conceptual basis for first language acquisition. In R.L. Schiefelbusch and L.L. Lloyd (Eds.): *Language Perspectives—Acquisition, Retardation and Intervention.* Baltimore, Md.: University Park Press, 1974.

Crystal, D., Fletcher, P., and Garmen, M.: *The Grammatical Analysis of Language Disability: A Procedure for Assessment and Remediation.* London, England: Edward Arnold (Publishers) Ltd., 1976.

DeVilliers, P. and DeVilliers, J.: Early judgments of semantic and syntactic acceptability by children. *Journal of Psycholinguistic Research, 1,* 299-310, 1972.

Dunn, L.M., Smith, J.O., and Horton, K.: Peabody Language Development Kits. Circle Pines, Minn.: America Guidance Services, 1965.

Engelmann, S. and Osborn, J.: *Distar.* Chicago, Ill.: Science Research Associates, 1972.

Feldman, C.F. and Rodgon, M.: *The Effects of Various Types of Adult Responses in the Syntactic Acquisition of Two- and Three-Year-Olds.* Departmnt of Psychology, University of Chicago, 1970.

Fraser, C., Bellugi, U., and Brown, R.: Control of grammar in imitation, comprehension, and production. *Journal of Verbal Learning and Verbal Behavior, 2,* 121-135, 1963.

Gray, B. and Ryan, B.: *Gray-Ryan Program for the Non-Language Child.* Champaign, Ill.: Research Press, 1973.

Lee, L.: *Developmental Sentence Analysis.* Evanston, Ill.: Northwestern

62   *Speech/Language Clinician's Handbook*

University Press, 1974.

Lee, L., Koeningsknecht, R., and Mulhern, S.: *Interactive Language Development Teaching.* Evanston, Ill.: Northwestern University Press, 1975.

Leonard, L.: *Meaning in Child Language.* New York, N.Y.: Grune and Stratton, 1977.

McNeill, D.: *The Acquisition of Language: The Study of Developmental Psycholinguistics.* New York, N.Y.: Harper and Row, 1970.

Menyuk, P.: A preliminary evaluation of grammatical capacity of children. *Journal of Verbal Learning and Verbal Behavior, 2,* 429-349, 1963.

Ruder, K. and Hermann, P.: Imitation and comprehension procedures in establishment of a second language in first and second graders. Research Progress Report, Bureau of Child Research Laboratory, University of Kansas, Lawrence, 1973.

Ruder, K., Smith, M., and Hermann, P.: Effects of verbal imitation and comprehension training on verbal production of lexical items. In L.V. McReynolds (Ed.): *Developing Systematic Procedures for Training Children's Language.* American Speech and Hearing Association Monograph, 18, Danville, Ill.: Interstate Press, 1974.

Slobin, D. and Welsh, C.A.: Elicited imitation as a research tool in developmental psycholinguistics. In C. Lavatelli (Ed.): *Language Training in Early Childhood Education.* Urbana, Ill.: University of Illinois Press, 1971.

Waryas, C. and Ruder, K.: On the limitations of language comprehension procedures and an alternative. *Journal of Speech and Hearing Disorders, 39,* 44-52, 1974.

Wiig, E.H. and Semel, E.M.: *Language Disabilities in Children and Adolescents.* Columbus, Ohio: Charles E. Merrill Publishing Co., 1976.

Chapter 3

LANGUAGE INTERVENTION TECHNIQUES FOR MENTALLY RETARDED CHILDREN

MARY ELLEN BRANDELL

STUDENT CLINICIANS presently enrolled in training programs will most likely be exposed to children with severe speech and language deficits. The clinician will probably be expected to assess the language skills of a severely retarded child, develop appropriate goals, plan an effective intervention program, and work with this individual under supervision in a clinical setting or in a public school classroom during a student teaching experience. Only in recent years has attention been focused on this special population.

It is no longer unusual for the public school therapist to have a number of severely or moderately retarded children in a regular case load. The speech pathologist may spend anywhere from four to forty hours per week in centers or classrooms designed specially for the developmentally disabled child. Until recently, efforts in dealing with the speech and language problems of the retarded have been relatively unproductive. Much of the intervention focused on behaviors such as inadequate memory span, poor attending skills, or inappropriate social behavior. Language therapy generally consisted of activities centered around vocabulary drills, sequencing tasks, or auditory discrimination programs. Results of these techniques were difficult to assess. It was not possible to collect data and account for any progress that a child may have made over a certain period of time.

The contributions to the areas of speech pathology and audiology from Bloom (1970), Brown (1973), McNeill (1970), and

Menyuk (1972) in the area of normal language development have added new dimensions of intervention procedures with retarded children. Knowledge concerning development of speech and language skills in the normal child has given us more tools to use in assessing the child with deficient speech and language skills and planning a program based on the results from the evaluation.

The first conference conducted specifically to provide information to professions responsible for clinical services to improve the speech and language of mentally retarded children was held in Kansas City, Missouri in February, 1970. This was sponsored by the Children's Bureau, Social Rehabilitation Services, Department of Health, Education and Welfare. Two more conferences followed during that year, which were designed to help clinicians gain some perspective in the complex area of language and to present information about the programs that were available to mentally retarded children throughout the country. Significant contributions were made by McLean (1973), Miller and Yoder (1973), and Kent, Klien, Falk, and Guenther (1973) regarding intervention programs. These techniques have proven to be successful with the mentally retarded population.

The Education for all Handicapped Children Act (Public Law 94-142), which states that all speech handicapped children between the ages of three and twenty-one years must be provided with necessary services, has increased the need for more speech pathologists with the skills to work with this population. The present policies in most states encourage the placement of mentally retarded children in a day school program and a normal home environment rather than an institutional setting. In the State of Michigan, for example, the number of children presently living in Regional Centers for the Developmentally Disabled has been cut by more than 50 percent in the last five years. In some instances, children living in these centers are transported to neighborhood schools each day and integrated as much as possible with normal children, but spend part of the day in special rooms designed to meet their unique needs.

Public Law 94-142 states that the speech pathologist must not only provide services to the child with deficient language skills, but also develop appropriate objectives based on diagnostic data.

The objectives for remediation must also contain the time frame in which the intervention will be conducted and the criteria that must be reached before the objectives can be considered to be accomplished.

This chapter has been written to provide the speech clinician with techniques to use in the assessment and intervention of language problems with the mentally retarded child.

ASSESSMENT TECHNIQUES

Before a clinician begins to develop an intervention program, the child's current level of language functioning must be determined. The results of an evaluation can serve as a baseline for therapy, providing appropriate tests are used. When a clinician is asked to serve children enrolled in a trainable mentally retarded classroom, it can be assumed that all of the children will be deficient in one or more language areas. Testing should not be done to determine whether the child is functioning below the norms established for his age level. Rather, tests that can give the clinician information regarding specific areas for intervention should be used. Occasionally, a clinician will identify a child who has been misdiagnosed; however, this is usually a rare occurrence.

Any initial assessment should include an audiological evaluation. Both pure tone and impedance testing should be included in the examination. Language delay can be facilitated by intermittent middle ear pathology. Studies conducted with mentally impaired adult populations and normal preschool children support this theory, e.g. Seestedt and Brandell (1976), Brandell and Seestedt (1977), Holmes and Kunze (1975). In each of these studies, a high incidence of middle ear pathology was found in the MR population. There was also a high correlation between middle ear problems identified by impedance testing and language delay. This included both expressive and receptive skills. The mentally retarded child should be seen annually for a routine audiological examination.

Miller (1978) views the assessment process as containing some basic components that include the establishment of baseline functioning. Within these parameters, the developmental level of the child can be determined and the behaviors needing remediation can be specified. These basic components also allow for an opportunity to measure the behavioral change that may be used in assessing children's language behavior: standardized tests, non-standardized tests, developmental scales, and behavioral observation.

The next section of this chapter will focus on specific assessment tools and methods, which can effectively assess the language behavior of the mentally retarded child. Results of the efficacy of these measures can be found in the literature and can be documented as appropriate diagnostic procedures and used in writing the annual IEP (Individual Education Plan).

Standardized Methods

Standardized tests are usually the most difficult to use effectively with the moderately or the severely mentally impaired child because of the distractibility and poor attending behaviors of these children. Most of the diagnostic tools used routinely by speech clinicians are designed for the normal child. The Receptive-Expressive Emerging Language Test (Bzoch and League, 1971) is standardized and lends itself to be administered to the mentally retarded child. There are no time limitations, and the test can be given in an informal manner. The clinician may also use a parent to help with the assessment. The Utah Test of Language Development (Mecham, Jex, & Jones, 1967) is a formal assessment procedure and can be used with children with limited expressive skills. The Test for Auditory Comprehension of Language (Carrow, 1974) can be used successfully with the child whose speech intelligibility is poor. This test also yields information that is beneficial for the clinician in planning a remediation program. The TACL can also be useful for the older mentally impaired youth or adult. A token or edible reinforcement system works well in administering this test to a highly distractible child. It is limited to assessing only comprehension skills. A test that is used in residential and regional centers to evaluate large numbers of retarded children over a short period of time is the Verbal Language Development Scale (Mecham, 1971). It covers broad areas and is not specific enough to assist the clinician in developing an adequate remediation plan with the results. However, it does have a score sheet and gives an age range of functioning ability. The language sample yields much information about the child's expressive abilities and is the most powerful diagnostic tool the clinician can use. The results of the language sample can be analyzed according to a model such as the one developed by Roger Brown (1973) and presented as a standard assessment measure. The level or stage of language functioning and the score generated by computing the Mean Length of Utterance can be used effectively for planning a language program, as a baseline before initiating therapy and as an assessment to measure the effectiveness of a program. Results of the language sample can also be used in writing the annual IEP. Boxx (1977) developed a handbook that outlines effective ways to collect, analyze, and interpret a language sample. For the clinician who may not be familiar with Roger Brown's Stages of Morphological Development, an illustration follows.

SUMMARY OF
BROWN'S STAGES OF MORPHOLOGICAL DEVELOPMENT (1973)

STAGE	SPAN OF MEAN LENGTH OF UTTERANCE	M/MLU	APPROXIMATE AGE
I	1.5–2.0	1.75	15–30 months
II	2.0–2.5	2.25	28–36 months
III	2.5–3.0	2.75	36–42 months
IV	3.0–3.7	3.50	40–46 months
V	3.7–4.5	4.00	42–52+ months

Developmental Order of *Acquisition* of grammatical morphemes

Earliest	Present progressive (Running, Walking) in, on plural (*s* and *z* markers)	Stage II
	past irregular (go, went, run, ran) possessive (boy's coat, mommy's shoe) uncontractible copula (This is pretty)	Stage III
	articles (a, an, the) past regular (jump, jumped, cry, cried) third person regular (boys walk)	Stage IV
Latest	third person irregular (boys have, boy does uncontractible auxiliary (Boys are walking) contractible copula (he's sick) contractible auxiliary (he's sleeping, he's running)	Stage V

"Stages" are determined by the child's MLU (*m*ean *l*ength of *u*tterance)

While the developmental order of acquisition is invariant, the age levels may vary considerably among children. Remember, these age levels are *only approximations*.

Nonstandardized Tests to Assess Language

There are a number of nonstandardized assessment approaches available to the speech pathologist. Leonard, Prutting, Perozzi, and Berkley (1978) have compiled a review of available approaches. Their work also includes a comprehensive bibliography of nonstandard assessment techniques. The purpose of their publication is to provide a justification for the use of nonstandard tests as a necessary supplement to standardized information. They view this as necessary to plan an effective intervention program. Receptive and expressive measures as well as the construction of nonstandardized measures are included in this publication.

The Environmental Language Inventory (MacDonald & Nichols, 1974) gives a comprehensive assessment of the developmentally delayed child. It also provides the clinician with useful information to assist in planning therapy. Sevener (1973) developed the Receptive and Expressive Language Assessment for Young or Developmentally Delayed Children. This assessment includes tasks to test the child's comprehension of object function, ability to follow commands and imitate motor skills, as well as examining his core vocabulary (verbs, nouns, and prepositions). The Modified Language Acquisition Program Final Tests (Kent, Klien, Faulk, and Guenther, 1972) was designed for the retarded child and was meant to be accompanied by the testing and training procedures described in *A Modified Language Acquisition Program for use by Attendants and Attendant-Supervised Retarded Trainer-Student Pairs* (Rowland, 1972). The child's performance in attending skills, motor and vocal imitation, and expressive and receptive language are assessed. Evaluation of Cognitive Behavior in Young Nonverbal Child (Chappell & Johnson, 1976) suggests ways in which the speech clinician can determine whether nonspeaking children are failing to learn in general or are failing to learn verbal competence. The authors relate verbal development to object knowledge development at three sequential levels of use in evaluation. Examples of behavior patterns at each level are provided, and an approach to promote the child's cognitive response to familiar household objects is suggested. This assessment can be very helpful to the clinician. A record form for observation is included in the publication.

Developmental Scales

Most currently published checklists are based upon standardized scales. The Portage Guide to Early Education (Shearer et al., 1974) comes in two parts: (1) A Checklist of Behaviors and (2) a Card File containing curriculum ideas. The checklist was developed by identifying behaviors from a variety of preschool developmental scales and tests. Four areas can be assessed with this instrument: Cognition, Self-Help, Motor Skills, and Language. The Checklist and Card File can aid in assessing present behavior, targeting emerging behavior, and then help the speech clinician to provide techniques of how to train each behavior. The Communicative Evaluation Chart (Anderson, 1963) is a means by which a clinician can gain an impression of a child's abilities and/ or disabilities in language and performance. Language items deal with coordination of the speech musculature, development of hearing acuity and auditory perception, acquisition of vowels and consonants, and development of receptive and expressive skills. This checklist was designed to be used as a screening tool, but can be an effective instrument for the "difficult to test child." The Telstar Developmental Checklist (Authier, Klerekoper, & Cook, 1976) classifies growth in five general areas: physical, self-help, social, academic, and communication. The Telstar manual accompanies the checklist and includes some instructions for teaching the tasks, and also gives the criteria for scoring. The Telstar Checklist represents correct sequences of development in sufficiently small steps so that it will be helpful in establishing baseline behavior. A Developmental Checklist, published by Wayne-Westland Michigan Public Schools Systems (1975), provides a detailed assessment guide for speech and language skills for the child through the twelve-year level. It includes the areas of Phonology, Morphology, Syntax, and Semantics. Specific examples of performance are given in each area. The checklist offers a guide to the speech clinician in developing remediation programs based on developmental norms.

Behavioral Observation

Clinical observation of the child may be the most important of all assessment techniques; however, it is often the most difficult area for the clinician to use effectively. It is common to read the following comments on diagnostic reports: "The child was frustrated," "The client acted extremely shy," "The youngster had a short attention span," or "He appeared to have emotional problems." Clinicians usually rely on superficial labeling rather than focus on observable behavior only. The behavior that is being assessed must be *observable* behavior. Harris and Schiefelbusch (1976) view the test for observability as follows: Can other persons see the same behavior at the same time? Do they all agree when the behavior did or did not occur? Do they agree on how many times it occurred and agree on the force or intensity with which it occurred? There must be agreement between other concerned persons as to what actually happened during the evaluation session.

One cannot measure "frustration" or "shyness." However, the clinician can record the number of times the child banged his head, refused to respond, sighed, put his hands over his face, or crawled under the table. The clinician must ask the question, "What behaviors did this child demonstrate that indicated that he was frustrated?"

Efforts to change behavior can be included in goals for management. Harris and Schiefelbusch include many forms in behavior change. The behavior may change in force. Does the child bang his head on the table so that he injures himself? The duration of a behavior may change. A child may put his hands over his face for five seconds or may hide his face for five minutes. The latency between a behavior and some event may also vary. The number of times a behavior occurs during a certain period of time may vary. Did the child crawl under the table every time his mother walked into the room? Did the child bang his head on the table ten times while the clinician was attempting to obtain a language sample and only once while he was putting a puzzle together?

Much information can be obtained by watching a child in a free play situation. Does the child throw the blocks around the room or does he attempt to build something or stack them? Does the child throw the toy dishes on the floor or does he set the table and play with the toy stove appropriately? How long does the child sit and stay with a task?

The clinician must be accountable for goals that have been developed in a management plan. If the goals include extinction of a behavior, the clinician must be sure that the behavior is observable and can be measured, and must devise a way to record the changes over a period of time.

PLANNING AN INTERVENTION PROGRAM

Articulation disorders occur in a higher incidence in mentally retarded children than in the normal population. However, the major deficit in the retarded child's communication skills is in limited and inadequate receptive and expressive language skills. Miller and Yoder (1972) concluded that mentally retarded children who do have language develop their language code in a manner similar to that of normal children but at a slower rate. The criteria for planning a management program should include the following:

1. A language training program should begin at the child's developmental level or linguistic stage as determined by speech and language assessments.
2. A management program should be based on an appropriate set of goals or language related behaviors. Long-range goals as well as short term behavioral objectives should be included.
3. The intervention program should be based on normal language acquisition.
4. The language program should include a systematic approach to help the child achieve more appropriate language skills.

The intervention techniques outlined in this chapter are designed for the verbal child.   Nonvocal systems will not be discussed.

Numerous programs have been used effectively with the mentally retarded child with very limited verbal skills. Training strategies developed by Kent (1973), Bricker, Ruder, and Vincent (1978), Love et al. (1974), and Stremel and Waryas (1974) include a prelinguistic phase. There will be a significant number of children who will not progress beyond the prelinguistic stage of development. They will be able to utilize minimal verbal skills; however, they will never be candidates for some of the structured programs discussed in this chapter. The next section will deal with skills that are necessary before placing a mentally retarded child in a structured language intervention program.

Training Prelinguistic Skills

Prelinguistic skills are usually acquired by the normal child by eighteen months. Prelinguistic training consists of teaching the child motor and verbal imitation, naming and labeling objects, and the symbolic functions of agent, action, and object.   The eighteen-month-old child communicates with a limited number of utterances. By handing his snowsuit to his mother and saying, "Go bye-bye," the youngster lets his mother know, "I want you to put on my snowsuit and take me outside for a walk."   Bloom (1970) and Brown (1973) describe these early two-word strings as expressing underlying semantic relations as possession (mine), recurrence (more milk), location (cookie here), and negation (no nite-nite) . The same semantic functions carry on throughout all stages of development and result in the adult language form. For example, a young child has acquired the concept of negation when he shakes his head when saying milk, indicating that he does not want any more milk to drink.

Schiefelbusch, Ruder, and Bricker (1977) view the following steps as antecedent to more complex learning phases and should be incorporated into the intervention plan:

1. To train the child to watch the actions of the clinician and to listen to verbal directions.
2. To train the child to sit appropriately during the instruc-

tion period and to handle the objects utilized in the clinical setting in an appropriate manner.

3. To imitate gestures and vocalizations from the clinician.
4. To learn the symbolic relationship between a spoken word and an object and the naming of several such objects.
5. To learn the words for the person who works with the child, the actions that are performed, and the objects that are present in the environment.

The programs discussed earlier in this chapter provide for the acquisition of entry behaviors such as attending skills, verbal imitation, motor imitation, and object naming. More emphasis should be placed upon the training of semantic relations at the prelinguistic stage. The clinician should be exposed to strategies that can be used as assessment techniques as well as training methods. The following represents an assessment method developed by Olsen (1977), which can also be used in a training program.

Function	Structure	Test of Underlying Function	Training of Underlying Function
		Concepts	Concept
1. Recurrence	More	Have child interact with a number of objects. Observe which objects are most attractive to him. Reintroduce these favorites to child and take them away from his view. Observe his desire to retrieve objects.	Clinician has bubble pipe and blows bubbles so that child can see; When clinician has the child's attention, stop the activity. When the child indicated by gesture or verbalizations (grunt) that he wants the clinician to continue, the clinician should first say, "More?" You want *more* bubbles?" Then repeat the sequence over again.
2. Nonexistence	all-gone Bye	Does child continue to look for an object you have just hidden.	Clinician takes a toy that child had been playing with and hides it while child watches.

Function	Structure	Test of Underlying Function	Training of Underlying Function
		Concepts	*Concept*
		Does child look for person who has left room e.g. mother. Turn off a TV set—say "all gone" (may be used in conjunction with "more"—turn TV back on when child used gestures or verbal production.	Clinician pairs his activity with "All gone." Clinician fills cup with water and pours it into the sink with the child watching the activity. Clinician pairs this action with "All gone."
3. Rejection	No	This is the semantic contrast of recurrence. Test is the same, except that some undesirable, such as vinegar, replaces the ice cream.	Show the child an ugly bug. Ask if he wants to see it again. Pick up child during play and require him to sit on clinician's lap for an extended period till he indicates he wants down; refuse this request by saying "No."
4. Agent	Subject of Sentence	(a) early test of this is observational. Does child indicate he recognizes initiators of actions, e.g. when a ball is thrown, does he return it to the experimenter to have the action repeated. (b) later tests can be more sophisticated using a match-to-sample format. Can child match an agent performing different actions when one of the choices is the same individual being the recipient of an action. That is, does the child discriminate be-	Have a set of dolls available and interact with the child by having the dolls perform actions, e.g. sit, walk, eat, etc.

Function	Structure	Test of Underlying Function	Training of Underlying Function
		Concepts	*Concept*
		tween the person giving and the person receiving.	
		Does child turn back to the source of sound after it ceases.	
5. Action	Verb	(a) early test of this is imitative. Can the child imitate some basic actions such as eat, throw, etc. which will be the focus of subsequent verb training.	Have the child imitate vocalizations or reaching for and touching body parts: ie. "See my eyes," "Touch your hair," etc.
		(b) more sophisticated test again involves match-to-sample format where the child is asked to match actions when agents and/or objects differ from those of the sample.	
		Is the child able to track or follow motion, e.g. have 2 mobiles, which are motor operated. Turn them on alternately Observe whether the child visually follows the mobile which is moving.	
6. Object		(a) early general test is again observational. Does child perform similar actions to dissimilar objects, e.g. he throws both a ball and a block.	Use toy dishes and pretend to eat and feed toy dolls or toy animals, etc. Try to get the child to imitate. Use toy stove and see if child will imitate cooking food, baking cake, etc.
		(b) match-to-sample test. Can child match two items when their only commonality is that they are recipients of	

Function	Structure	Test of Underlying Function	Training of Underlying Function
		Concepts	*Concept*
		actions, e.g. a *car* being pushed, being matched to boy being pushed, when other choices include a car involved in no action.	
		Have various objects available plus a can. See if the child will put the objects in a can. Next, observe what else he does with them. If he does nothing try to get him to imitate your actions (you use) object, he a different one.	
7. Possession	Mine	Will child pull a toy away from someone and bring toy to himself indicating mine. Take the child's coat, hat, or other possession away from him. Perhaps you could pretend to wear the item. Does the child indicate that it is his, and wants it back?	Get a favorite toy of the child's, take it away but put it in the child's view. When he attempts to retrieve it, encourage and assist him by saying "Yes, this is yours."
8. Attributive	Adjectives	(a) early test is simply a discrimination test of attributes being tested, e.g. color discrimination test, shape, size. (b) following discrimination test is a categorization test (match-to-sample format) e.g., can the child match colors which vary in shade of color.	Have a set of matching blocks varying in color. Assist the child in finding "another one" exactly like it. Matching objects and pictures may also be used.

Function	Structure	Test of Underlying Function	Training of Underlying Function
		Concepts	Concept
		(c) following the categorization test is a test of the child's ability to recognize color as a salient attribute of objects which vary in shape, size and content, e.g. can a child match toys of the same color category, when the type, size and shape of toys vary.	

LANGUAGE PROGRAMS FOR THE DEVELOPMENTALLY DISABLED CHILD

Many language training programs are available to the speech clinician and appropriate for intervention with the mentally retarded child (see References at the end of this chapter). Two programs, which can be used by inexperienced clinicians and follow normal language development principles, will be discussed in detail.

The first program to be presented was developed by Love, Miller, Otermat, and Perlrix (1974) at the Franklin County, Ohio Program for the Mentally Retarded. The program incorporates all the prelinguistic phases and includes models for objectives at each level. The following is an outline of the training model.

FRANKLIN COUNTY PROGRAM FOR THE MENTALLY RETARDED DEVELOPMENTAL LANGUAGE PROGRAM

Prerequisite Skills

I   Sitting
II   Eye Contact
III   Reaching for Objects
IV   Displacement of Objects
V   Motor Imitation with Objects

VI   Physical Imitation
VII   Mouth Imitation
VIII Sound Imitation

Presyntax
I   Relational Terms
      A Recurrence
      B Nonexistence
      C Disappearance
      D Rejection
      E Cessation
      F Existence
II   Substantives
      A nouns
      B actions
      C attributives
      D possession

Syntax Stage I A
I   Semantic Relations
      A Agent-Action
      B Action-Object
      C Agent-Object
      D Locatives
      E Possession
      F Questions by Inflection
II   Functional Relations
      A Recurrence
      B Nonexistence
      C Rejection
      D Denial

Syntax Stage I B
I   Three-Term Relations
      A Agent + Action + Object— (Boy sit chair)
      B Agent + Action + Location— (Boy walk home)
      C Action + Object + Location— (Walk boy home)
II   Noun Phrase Expansion

    A Attributive
    B Possessive
    C Recurrence
III   Four-Term Relations

Syntax Stage II

I   Noun Phrase
    A Determiners
       1. Demonstratives
       2. Quantifiers
       3. Possessive Pronouns
       4. Articles
    B Prepositions (in, on)
    C Plurals
II   Verb Phrase
    A Present Progressive (V + ing)
    B Catenative
III   Questions
    A Yes/No
    B Wh (wh + NP + doing/go) (what, where)
IV   Negation

Syntax Stage III

I   Noun Phrase Expansion
    A Det + Art + Adj + N
       M + N
       Pos + N ('s)
    B Prepositions
    C Indeterminers
    D Noun Plural
II   Verb Phrase
    A Irregular Past Tense
    B Uncontractible Copula
III   Auxiliaries
    A can't. don't _____V (don't walk)
    B do
IV   Negatives
    A NP + (neg) + VP

V   Yes/No Questions
   A Rising intonation
   B Nucelus = pronouns, (See my doggie?)
       modifiers, can't don't (You can't fix it?)
VI   Wh Questions
   A what
   B where
   C why

The second program presented in this chapter was designed by Allen and Brandell (1976) to be used with children and adults who were enrolled in educational settings in the Mt. Pleasant, Michigan public school district. Results of periodic assessment made over a two-year period indicated that this type of intervention method facilitated expressive language skills in a moderate to severe, language impaired population. The structure of the programs developed by Gray and Ryan (1974) and Mecham (1974) was used as a model. The sequence of the structures to be trained followed Brown's (1973) developmental order of acquisition of grammatical morphemes.

Language Program for the Mentally Retarded
Rationale for the Development of the MR Language Program

This program was developed in an attempt to fulfill the following requirements:

1. A structured program using token reinforcement had been successful in the past with both adult and child trainable MR's who were not in an institutionalized living situation. This was to be such a program, and hopefully as effective as the Monterey Language Program (1971), which was used in the past (Bihum and Brandell, 1975).
2. The program could be learned quickly so that the minimum of clinician training would be necessary.
3. It would follow a normal language development scale (Brown, 1973) in order of its individual units.
4. It would be a program that could be used in a training program to provide more stable continuation of therapy when new student clinicians were assigned to clients at the end of each term.

Design of the Program

The program is divided into two levels called Sections. Section I is titled Basic Language. Basic Language begins with one-word utterances (Nouns and Verbs) and extends through three-word Agent-Action-Object strings that contain no transformations.

Section II contains all programs that require transformations, including the present progressive, regular past tense, and plurality. The presentation of all structures follows Brown's Acquisition of Morphemes.

All units use three levels of stimulus, and thus response difficulty. These levels are Imitation, Delayed Imitation, and Spontaneous levels.

Example:

1 = Imitation, 2 = Delayed Imitation, 3 = Spontaneous, in all units in both sections of the program.

Reinforcement

Two types of reinforcement are used; social and nonedible tokens. Social reinforcement (verbal praise in the form of "Good," or "Nice work," etc.) is used for all correct and aided responses. The social reinforcement always *precedes* any token reinforcement.

Token reinforcement is nonedible and is used on a tapered reinforcement schedule. Initially during a level of a unit, 100 percent of all correct responses will be reinforced with a token. When the client reaches a 70 percent correct response criterion level, token reinforcement schedule is reduced to 75 percent; that is, three out of four correct responses will be reinforced with tokens. When the client reaches a 90 percent correct criterion level, the reinforcement schedule becomes 50 percent token reinforcement (1 out of 2 responses are given token reinforcement). To move from one level to another *within a unit* (example: from 1 to 2, or −2 to −3), a client must have 10 consecutive correct responses at the 50 percent reinforcement level. When the new level is begun, the reinforcement schedule also begins at the beginning with 100 percent token reinforcement. To start a new unit, the client must have 20 consecutive responses at the 50 percent reinforcement schedule. This is the spontaneous (3) level only. A secondary token is received for 35 correct reinforced responses.

Recording the Data

Each response is recorded on a record sheet, and graphs of progress within a unit are kept. The following code is suggested.

+ = correct, social and token reinforced.

− = correct, with social reinforcement only.

√ = incorrect, nonreinforced response.

A = aided correct response: Assisted by the clinician and reinforced by social and token reinforcement, but not counted as correct toward reaching criterion.

Presentation of the Program

The program should be used for approximately 10 minutes per therapy session. For one or two minutes during each session, spontaneous speech should be encouraged by using a picture (s) from outside the program, which will provide opportunities to use the structures trained that day. Only social reinforcement will be used during this time, and leading questions to elicit responses may be used. It is a "spontaneous speech time" and is to be done every therapy session regardless of where a client is in a unit at that time. The type of responses made during this spontaneous speech time should be noted. By the time a client is approaching the criterion of 20 consecutive correct responses in the "spontaneous speech time" at the end of the session.

Specific Directions for Presentation

1. The following materials are needed:

   Picture Stimuli (pictures have been developed for this program) (see Appendix A)

   Score Sheet

   Token Reinforcements

   Container for Tokens

   Secondary Reinforcers (stickers, etc.)

2. Timing is important for maintaining the client's interest, as well as for eliciting a high number of responses per session.

This may also be called "pacing." Present the stimuli and, immediately after a correct response, give verbal reinforcement while simultaneously marking the score sheet with the writing hand and putting down the used picture with the other hand. Next, quickly place token in container (if response was correct or aided). Then promptly pick up the next picture and present the stimulus.

3. Let the client see only one picture at a time. Place all others face down. The verbal stimuli may be written on the backs of the pictures.

4. Whether the token is placed by the clinician or client in the container will depend on several factors, such as the motivation level of the client, distractibility, and the speech with which the client will reward himself.

5. If there is more than one item in a picture, the clinician should point to the one that is included in the response.

6. Any response that is semantically correct is marked as correct. Example: *cat* for *dog, Mom* for *lady,* etc. The only exception is if the client is working on building specific vocabulary.

Level I: Imitation

1. Present the verbal stimulus of "Name, say Verbal Stimulus," simultaneously presenting picture.

Example: "Mary, say 'dog biting boy.' "

Aided responses may consist of repeats, or extra verbal prompts ("Mary, look at this picture and say . . .") or expanding the client's inadequate response and having it imitated again. ("Mary, say 'biting,'" clinician may add "Good, Mary, but say the whole thing, 'dog biting boy,'" etc.) Remember that an aided response is reinforced if correct, but is not counted toward criterion. If the client does not give a correct response, mark incorrect.

Level II: Delayed Imitation

With the *back* of the picture toward the client, present the verbal stimulus of "Name, when I show you the picture, say '. . . (verbal stimulus.)'" Wait 3 to 5 seconds, and then turn the picture around and have client response.

If the clinician has trouble making the client wait to respond until the picture is turned, the following techniques may be used.

Shorten the waiting time, and then, as the client gradually begins to succeed, gradually lengthen the waiting time to the required 3 to 5 seconds. Do not count criterion for this level as reached until it is reached at the correct delay time. The second technique is to use the hand signals "stop" (palm of hand facing client) and "speak" (motioning a type of "come" response) after the signs have been explained. The verbal command "wait" may also be used if the client begins to speak too soon.

Aided responses are responses similar to level I. Thus, direct imitation following a repeat of stimulus can be used and counted as an aided response.

Level III: Sponetaneous

The picture is shown, and a verbal stimulus to elicit a spontaneous response is presented. It is of the type "Mary, What is happening here?" "Where is the dog?"; "What is the boy doing?", etc. Each unit will suggest a stimulus probe item.

Aided responses may consist of "Say the whole thing" if a partial response is given, or again presenting an item to be imitated.

Section I: Basic Verbal Language

LEVELS	STRUCTURE TO BE TRAINED	STIMULUS	DESIRED RESPONSE
1	Basic Nouns Imitation	"Say (dog) ."	Single noun, e.g. "dog"
2	Basic Nouns Delayed	"When I show you the picture, say (noun) ."	Single noun, e.g. "house"
3	Basic Nouns Spontaneous	"What is this ?"	Single noun, e.g. "Cat"

2

LEVELS	STRUCTURE TO BE TRAINED	STIMULUS	DESIRED RESPONSE
1	Basic Verbs Imitation	"Say (verb) ."	Single Verb, e.g. "bite"
2	Basic Verbs Delayed	"When I show you the picture, say ."	Single Verb, e.g. "walk"
3	Basic Verbs Spontaneous	"What is (noun) doing?"	Single Verb, e.g. "sleep"

3

LEVELS	STRUCTURE TO BE TRAINED	STIMULUS	DESIRED RESPONSE
1	Two word Agent + Action	"Say (boy walk .)"	Agent + Action, e.g. "boy walk"
2	Agent + Action Delayed	"When I show you the picture say (agent + action)."	Agent + Action, e.g. "girl cry"
3	Agent + Action Spontaneous	"What is (agent) doing?"	Agent + Action, e.g. "boy sleep"

4

LEVELS	STRUCTURE TO BE TRAINED	STIMULUS	DESIRED RESPONSE
1	Action + Object Imitation	"Say (carry dog) ."	Action + Object, e.g. "carry dog"
2	Action + Object Delayed	"When I show you the picture, say (action + agent) ."	Action + Object, e.g. "carry dog" Action + Action,
3	Action + Object Spontaneous	"What is Agent doing?"	e.g. "boy carry dog"

5

LEVELS	STRUCTURE TO BE TRAINED	STIMULUS	DESIRED RESPONSE
1	3 word Agent + Action + Object Imitation	"Say (agent + action + object) ."	Agent + Action + Object, e.g. "boy carry dog"
2	Agent + Action + Object Delayed	"When I show you the picture say (agent + action + object ."	Agent + Action + Object, e.g. "girl kick ball"
3	Agent + Action + Object Spontaneous	"What is Agent doing?"	Agent + Action + Object, e.g. "lady carry baby"

Section II: Transformations

LEVELS	STRUCTURE TO BE TRAINED	STIMULUS	DESIRED RESPONSE
1	2 word present progressive imitation	Picture plus verbal model	Agent + Action + ing e.g. "boy running"
2	2 word present progressive, delayed imitation	Picture, verbal model and delay	Agent + Action + ing e.g. "boy kicking"
3	2 word present progressive spontaneous	Picture + "What is agent doing?"	Agent + Action + ing e.g. "lady eating dinner"

2

LEVELS	STRUCTURE TO BE TRAINED	STIMULUS	DESIRED RESPONSE
1	3 word present progressive imitation	Picture plus verbal model	Agent + Action + ing + Object, e.g. "dog biting boy"
2	3 word present progressive delayed imitation	Picture + Verbal Model + Time delay	Agent + Action + ing + Object, e.g. "boy opening door"
3	3 word present progressive: spontaneous	Picture + "What is Agent doing?"	Agent + Action + ing e.g. "man driving car" + Object,

3

LEVELS	STRUCTURE TO BE LEARNED	STIMULUS	DESIRED RESPONSE
3	"in" + Object	"Where is the agent?"	"in" + Object, e.g. "in box"
3	Agent + "in" + Object	"Where is the agent?"	Agent + "in" + Object, e.g. "boy in house"
3	(Optional) 4 word "in"	"Where is the agent?"	Agent + Action + "in" + Object e.g. "boy swimming in water"

4

LEVELS	STRUCTURE TO BE LEARNED	STIMULUS	DESIRED RESPONSE
3	"on" + Object	"Where is the agent?"	"in" + Object, e.g. "on car"
3	Agent + "on" + Object	"Where is the agent?"	Agent + "on" + Object, e.g. "cat on car"
3	(Optional) 4 word "on"	"Where is the agent?"	Agent + Action + "on" + Object, e.g. "boy sitting on chair"

5

LEVELS	STRUCTURE TO BE LEARNED	STIMULUS	DESIRED RESPONSE
3	Preposition + Present Progressive	"Where is the agent?"	Agent + Action + ing + in + Object, e.g. "man driving car in street"
3	Preposition + Present Progressive	"Where is the agent?"	Agent + Action + ing +on + Object e.g. "lady cooking dinner on stove"

6

LEVELS	STRUCTURE TO BE LEARNED	STIMULUS	DESIRED RESPONSE
3	Plural Object + "s"	"What are these?"	Agent + "s," e.g. "shoes" (final position "s" must be present)
3	(Optional) Adjective + Agent + s (plural)	"What are these?"	Adjective + Agent + "s," e.g. "red shoes"

7

LEVELS	STRUCTURE TO BE LEARNED	STIMULUS	DESIRED RESPONSE
3	2 word irregular past tense; Agent + Action	"What did agent do yesterday?"	Agent + irregular past action, e.g. "boy stood"
3	3 word irregular past; Agent + Action + Object	"What did agent do yesterday?"	Agent + irregular past + Object, e.g. "lady ate food"

8

LEVELS	STRUCTURE TO BE LEARNED	STIMULUS	DESIRED RESPONSE
3	2 word possessive agent + "s" + Object	"Who's object is that?"	Agent + "s" + Object, e.g. "boy's shoes"
3	3 word possessive agent + "s" + adj. + Object	"Who's object is that?"	Agent + "s" + adj. + Object, e.g. "lady's big shoes"

9

LEVELS	STRUCTURE TO BE LEARNED	STIMULUS	DESIRED RESPONSE
3	3 word copula Agent + is + Action + ing	"What is agent doing?"	Agent + is + action + ing, e.g. "boy is standing"

10

LEVELS	STRUCTURE TO BE LEARNED	STIMULUS	DESIRED RESPONSE
3	Article "the" may be added to units 6, 7, 8	Depends on unit "the" is used with.	Response depends on unit used.

11

LEVELS	STRUCTURE TO BE LEARNED	STIMULUS	DESIRED RESPONSE
3	2 word regular past: Agent + Action + "ed"	"What did agent do yesterday?"	Agent + Action + ed, e.g. "boy carried"

LEVELS	STRUCTURE TO BE LEARNED	STIMULUS	DESIRED RESPONSE
3	3 word regular past Agent + Action + ed + Object	"What did agent do yesterday?"	Agent + Action + ed + Object, e.g. "boy carried dog"

12

LEVELS	STRUCTURE TO BE LEARNED	STIMULUS	DESIRED RESPONSE
3	2 word third person regular	"What does the agent do?"	Agent + Action + "s," e.g. "boy carried"
3	2 word third person regular Agent + Action + "S" + Object	"What does the agent do?"	Agent + Action + "s" + Object, e.g. "boy carries dog"

13

LEVELS	STRUCTURE TO BE LEARNED	STIMULUS	DESIRED RESPONSE
3	Pronouns "He" 3 word he + action + Object	"What does man/boy do?"	"He" + Action + Object e.g. "He eat(s) food"

14

LEVELS	STRUCTURE TO BE LEARNED	STIMULUS	DESIRED RESPONSE
3	Pronoun "she" 3 word She + Action + Object	"What does lady/girl do?"	"She" + Action + Object, e.g. "She eats food"

15

LEVELS	STRUCTURE TO BE LEARNED	STIMULUS	DESIRED RESPONSE
3	He-She comparison 3 word "pronoun + Action + Object	"What does agent do?"	"He/She" + Action + Object, e.g. "He kicks ball" Use pictures of males as well as females so selection of pronouns is necessary.

16

LEVELS	STRUCTURE TO BE LEARNED	STIMULUS	DESIRED RESPONSE
3	Possessive pronoun "his" 2 word	"Who's object is that?"	"His" + Object, e.g. "His dog"

17

LEVELS	STRUCTURE TO BE LEARNED	STIMULUS	DESIRED RESPONSE
3	Possessive Pronoun "Her," a word	"Who's object is that?"	Her + Object, e.g. "Her food"

Conclusion

The purpose of this chapter is to assist the clinician working with those children and adults who have severe language deficiencies. This is a special population with unique problems, which has not been effectively served in the past.

Efforts must continue to develop management methods that, facilitate language skills in the mentally retarded population. Professionals in the field of speech pathology and audiology have made significant contributions during the past decade. Results of their efforts can be seen in the achievements of a population that once was isolated in institutions.

References

Allen, S. and Brandell, M.E.: "Language Program for the Mentally Retarded." Paper presented at the Michigan Speech and Hearing Association Fall Convention, Boyne Mountain, Oct., 1976.

Anderson, R.: 1963, *Communication Evaluation Chart.* Cambridge, Educator's Publishing Service, 1963.

Authier, G., Klerekoper, P., and Cook, P.: Telestar Developmental Checklist, Alpena-Montmorency-Alvona Intermediate School District, Box 497, Alpena, Michigan 49707 (1976).

Bihum, V. and Brandell, M.E.: "A Comparison of Trainable Mentally Retarded Children and Adult Groups Utilizing the Monterey Language Program." Unpublished Independent Study, Central Michigan University, Mt. Pleasant, Michigan, 1975.

Bloom, L.: *Language Development: Form and Function in Emerging Grammars.* Cambridge, MIT Press, 1970.

Boxx, J.: "Methods for Collecting a Language Sample and a Model for Intervention." Second Annual Speech Clinician's Workshop, Central Michigan University, Mt. Pleasant, Michigan, May, 1977.

Brandell, M.E. and Seestedt, L.: "Language Delay and Middle Ear Pathology in a Headstart Population." Paper presented at Michigan Speech and Hearing Association Convention, Lansing, Michigan, Fall, 1977.

Bricker, D., Ruder, K., and Vincent, L.: "An Intervention Strategy for Language Deficient Children." In R.L. Schiefelbusch (Ed.): *The Basis of Language Intervention.* Baltimore, University Park Press, 1978.

Brown, R., *A First Language: The Early Stages.* Cambridge, Harvard University Press (1973).

Bzoch, K. and League, R.: *Receptive-Expressive Emergent Language Scale.* Gainesville, Florida, Anhenja Press, 1971.

Chappell, G. and Johnson, G.: "Evaluation of Cognitive Behavior in the

Young Nonverbal Child." *Language Speech and Hearing Services in the Schools, VII:*6-16, 1976.

Carrow, E.:   Test for Auditory Comprehension of Language.   Austin, Learning Concepts, 1974.

Downing, L.:   *The Appropriateness of Language Programs with the Educable Mentally Retarded.*   Southwest Texas State University, 1975.

Gray, B. and Ryan, B.:   *A Language Program for the Non-Language Child.*   Champaign, Research Press, 1973.

Harris, N. and Schiefielbusch, R.:   *Teaching Special Children.*   New York, McGraw-Hill Publishing Co., 1976.

Holmes, V. and Kunze, L.:   Effect of chronic otitis media on language and speech development.   *Pediatrics, 43,* 833-839, 1969.

Holton, J., Goman, T., and Lent, C.:   *Emerging Language Communication Skill Builders.*   P.O. Box 4081, Tucson, Arizona 85733, 1975.

Kent, L.:   *A Language Program for Severely Retarded Children.*   Kalamazoo, Western Michigan University Press, 1973.

Kent, L., Klien, D., Falk, A. and Guenther, H.:   "The Modified Language Acquisition Program Final Tests."   In McLean, J., Yoder, D., and Schiefelbusch, R. (Ed.):   *Language Intervention with the Retarded: Developing Strategies.*   Baltimore: University Park Press, 1972.

Leonard, L., Prutting, C.A., Perozzi, J.A., and Berkley, R.K.:   Non standardized approaches to the assessment of language behaviors.   *ASHA, 20,* 371-379, 1978.

Love, R., Miller, S., Otermat, C., and Perlrix, J.:   *Developmental Language Program.*   Franklin County Program for the Mentally Retarded, 1000 Kenniar Road, Columbus, Ohio 43212, 1974.

MacDonald, J. and Nichols, M.:   *Environmental Language Inventory.*   The Nisonger Center, Ohio State University, Ohio, 1974.

McLean, J.:   "Developing Clinical Strategies for Language Intervention with Mentally Retarded Children."   In McLean, J., Yoder, D., and Schiefelbusch, R. (Eds.):   *Language Intervention with the Retarded: Developing Strategies.*   Baltimore, University Park Press, 1973.

McNeill, D.:   *The Acquisition of Language: The Study of Developmental Psycholinguistics,* Chapter 9, New York, Harper and Row, 1970.

Mecham, M.:   *Motivation and Learning Centered Training Programs for Language Delayed Children.*   Salt Lake City, Word Making Productions, 1974.

Mecham, M.:   *Verbal Language Development Scale.*   Circle Pines, Minn., American Guidance Service, Inc., 1971.

Mecham, M.J., Jex, J., and Jones, D.:   *Utah Test of Language Development,* Communication Research Assoc., Box 11012 Salt Lake City, Utah, 1967.

Menyuk, P.:   *The Development of Speech.*   New York, Bobbs-Merrill, 1972.

Miller, J.:   "Assessing Children's Language Behavior: A Developmental

Process Approach." Presentation at Eighth Annual Conference on Communicative Disorders, Memphis, Tennessee, Febuary 22-25, 1978.

Miller, J. and Yoder, D.: "A Syntax Teaching Program" In McLean, J., Yoder, D., and Schiefelbusch, R. (Eds.): *Language Intervention with the Retarded: Developing Strategies.* Baltimore, University Park Press, 1973.

Miller, J.F. and Yoder, D.E.: "An ontogenetic Language Teaching Strategy for Retarded Children." In Lloyd, L.L. and Schiefelbusch, R.R. (Eds): *Language Perspectives: Acquisition, Retardation and Intervention.* Baltimore, University Park Press, 1974.

Mykelbust, H.: *Auditory Disorders in Children, A manual for differential diagnosis.* New York, Grune and Stratton, 1954.

Olsen, M.: "Informal Language Assessments." Presentation to Graduate Seminar, Central Michigan University, 1977.

Rowland, M.S.: *Modified Language Acquisition Program for use by Attendants and Attendant-Supervised Retarded Trainer-Student Pairs.* Michigan State University, Department of Elementary and Special Education, 1972.

Ruder, K.F.: Planning and programming for language intervention. In R.L. Schiefelbusch (Ed.): *The Bases of Language Intervention.* Baltimore, University Park Press, 1978.

Schiefelbusch, R., Ruder, K., and Bricker, W.: "Training Strategies for Language Deficient Children: An Overview." In Schiefelbusch, R. (Ed.): *The Bases of Languages Intervention, Baltimore,* University Park Press, 1977.

Seestedt, L. and Brandell, M.E.: "Incidence of Middle Ear Pathology in a Mentally Retarded Adult Population." Research Project, Central Michigan University, Mt. Pleasant, Michigan, 1976.

Sevenar, G.: "Receptive and Expressive Language Assessment for Young or Developmentally Delayed Children." UAF-Speech Pathology Kansas Center for Mental Retardation, University of Kansas, Lawrence, Kansas, 1973.

Shearer, D., Billingsley, J., Frohman, A., Hilliard, J., Johnson, F., and Shearer, M.: The Portage Guide to Early Education, Cooperative Educational Service Agency, Portage, Wisconsin 53901, 1974.

Stremel, K. and Waryas, C.: *A Behavioral-Psycholinguistic Approach to Language Training,* Bureau of Child Research. Universiy of Kansas, *ASHA* Monographs, 18, 1974.

Wayne-Westland, Michigan Public Schools, "Developmental Levels: A Checklist," 1975.

APPENDIX A

PICTURES ACCOMPANYING LANGUAGE PROGRAM
FOR THE MENTALY RETADED*

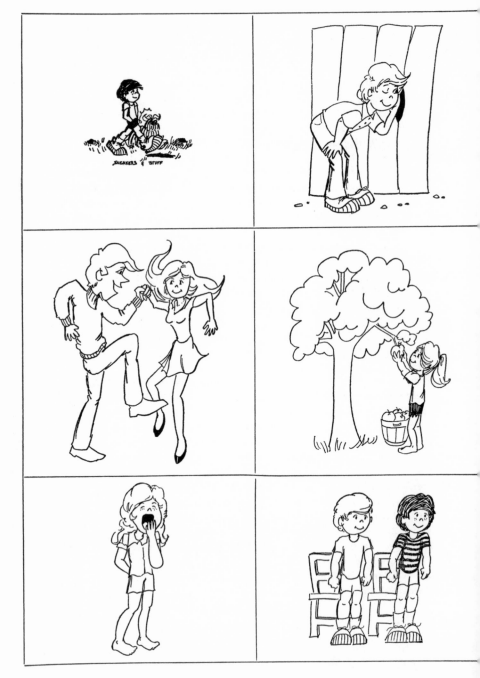

*Drawn by Penelope Faber, undergraduate student in Speech Pathology, Central Michigan University.

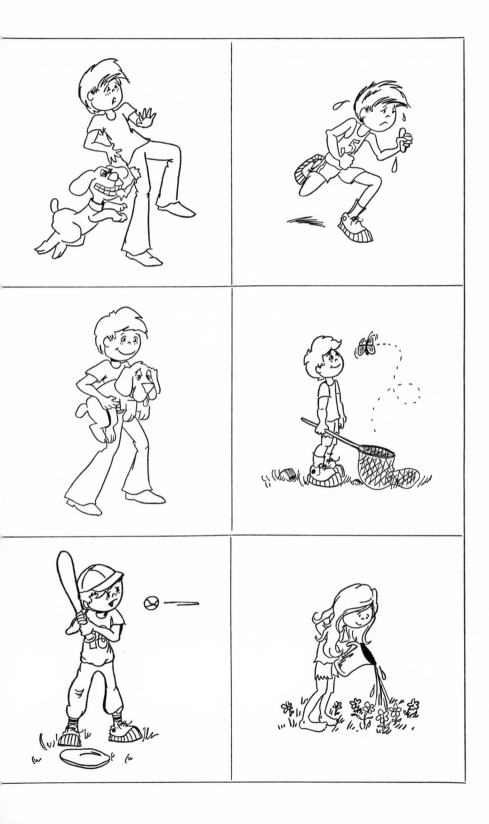

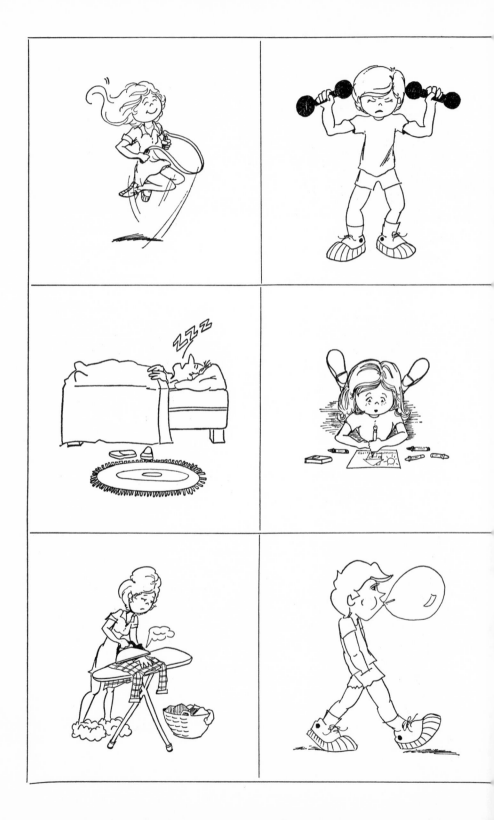

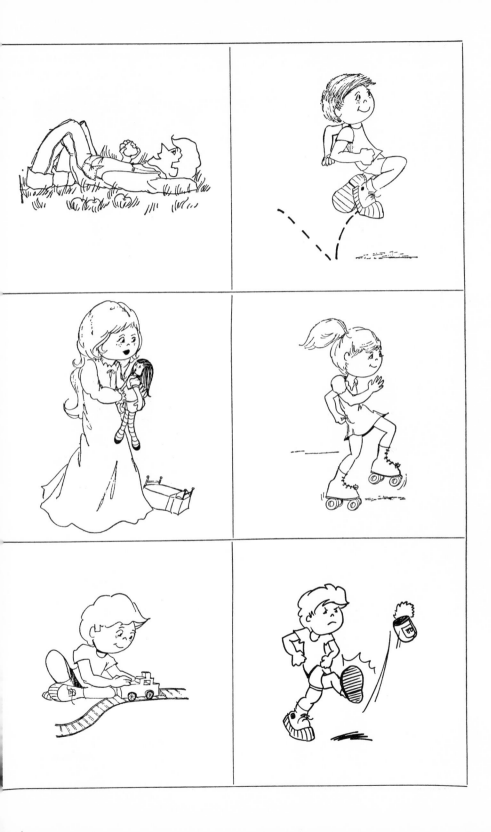

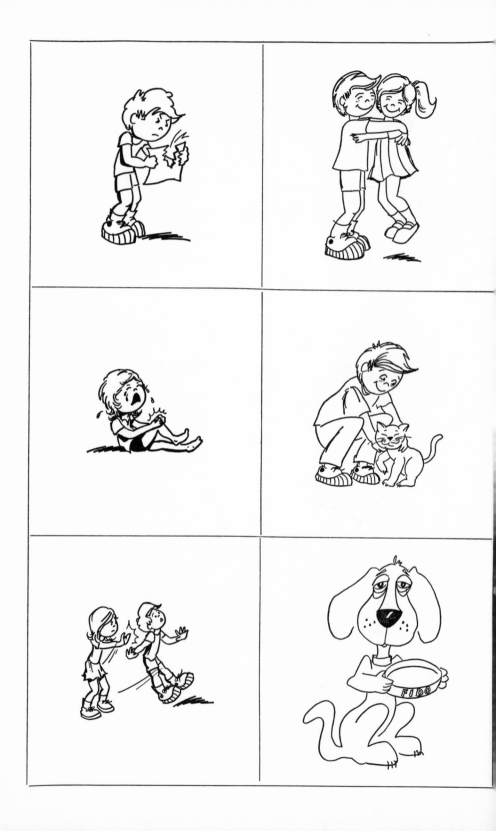

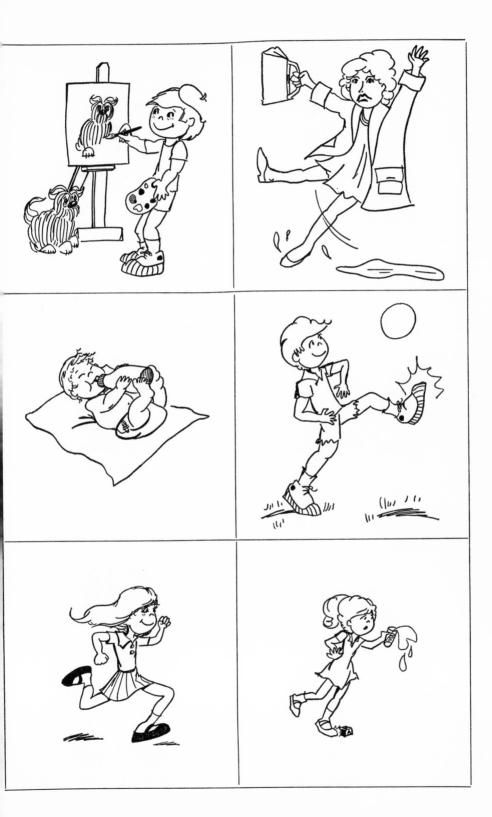

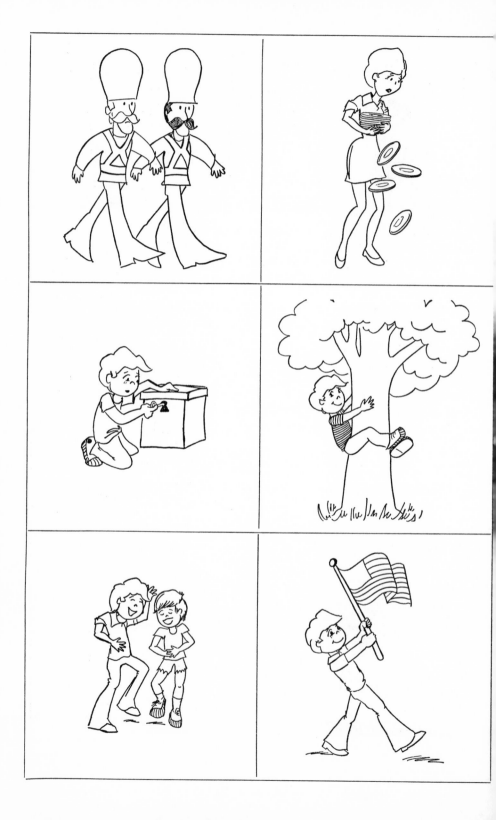

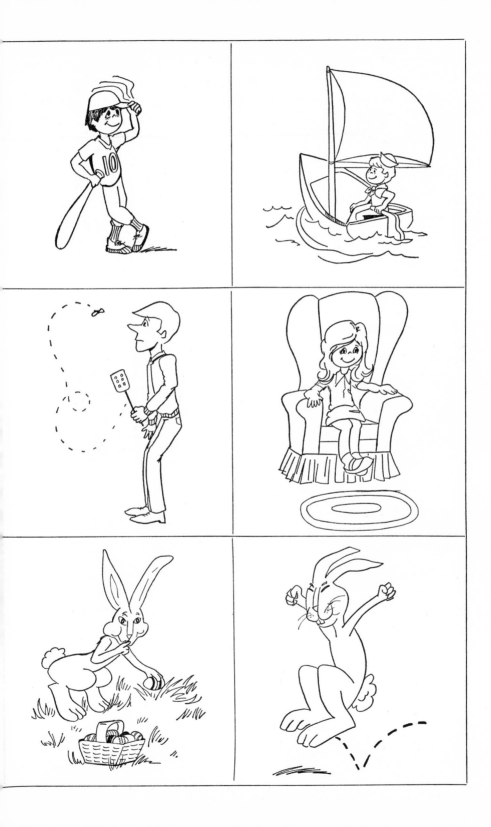

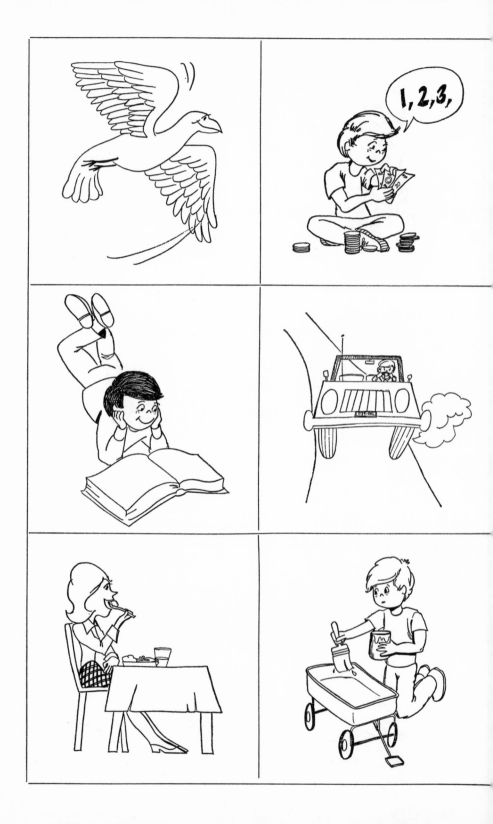

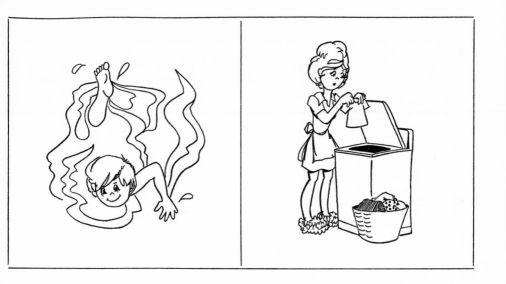

Chapter 4

FOREIGN DIALECTS

Constance Miller-Barnett

L EARNING A LANGUAGE is a very complex process involving an intricate system of rules. The young child amazingly accomplishes most of this feat by the age of four. The child's speech, or verbal language, carries unique properties resulting from the child's abilities and social experiences.

The foreign student learning American English as a second language has already developed a language unique to his culture. Consequently, a problem may occur when the native rule system is applied to English. [The sound system, meaning, word order, and intonation patterns of the student's native language may be quite different from the English system. A so-called "foreign accent" results when principles of other languages are applied to American English.]

Training of the English language for the foreign student involves the same major areas as seen in other therapy populations: language, articulation, fluency, and voice. The primary factor differentiating the foreign student is the already established first language, which at times may facilitate second language learning and at other times interfere. It is important for the therapist to determine some of the similarities and differences between the two languages to enhance the therapy process.

The ease with which a person learns a second language may be influenced by the age at which the second language is introduced. An infant born into a bilingual family or culture may experience little difficulty in developing both languages and may alternate the choice of language spoken according to the appropriate situation. However, if a child begins to learn a second language at the age of six or seven, the task becomes more difficult as the child has already established and reinforced usage of the first language. This may be influenced by what some authors term the "critical period" for language learning, which is thought to occur between the ages of zero to three years.

When working with the teenage or adult foreign person, simple materials should be used, which are not childlike. Structures should be trained at the appropriate level for that person. Also, the clinician should keep in mind that the foreign student is generally learning new ways of saying already acquired concepts rather than developing new concepts.

Diagnosis

As in all therapy processes, diagnosis is the first step toward remediation. With the foreign student, it is important to assess the client's language, articulation, fluency, and vocal intonation patterns.

Language Skills

Specifically, in terms of language assessment, both expressive and receptive abilities should be evaluated. A very helpful tool in determining the client's expressive skills is a language sample. A language sample consisting of about 100 consecutive spontaneous utterances may provide very useful information when analyzed for its phonological, morphological, syntactical, and semantic content. The Grammatic Closure subtest of the Illinois Test of Psycholinguistic Abilities (ITPA) (Kirk, McCarthy, and Kirk, 1968) or the use of nonsense sentences according to Berko's data (1961) may also provide valuable information as to the client's expressive use of morphological endings.

An overview of receptive language skills may be determined through the use of the Carrow Test of Auditory Comprehension of Language (1974) or the Assessment of Children's Language Comprehension (1969). Both of these tests encompass a variety of linguistic skills. Unfortunately, both are also geared for children and may be too childlike for the adult learning English as a second language. Receptive vocabulary should also be evaluated, and the Peabody Picture Vocabulary Test (Dunn, 1965) or Full-Range Picture Vocabulary Test (Ammons and Ammons, 1958) may provide insight concerning the client's skills in this area.

Articulation Assessment

Frequently, the foreign student experiences some difficulty in the articulation of English phonemes. Therefore, a thorough articulation test encompassing all phonemes, both consonants and vowels, should be given. The error sounds should then be deep tested to determine if the phonemes are produced correctly in any phonetic contexts. Those contexts articulated correctly during deep testing may be used as key words in therapy.

Related to the area of articulatory production is auditory discrimination. The foreign student may have difficulty detecting the difference between similar-sounding English words. This is especially true if the words contain phonemes not found in the foreign student's native language. Therefore, administration of a test for auditory discrimination may also provide some important diagnostic information.

Fluency Assessment

The fluency of an English speaker is greatly influenced by the stress and rhythm patterns used by a speaker. Stress, or accent, is important not only within words but also within sentences. It is also important to weaken the unstressed words and syllables. The native English speaker often accomplishes this feat by obscuring or reducing the vowels of unstressed syllables by substituting an /ə/ or /I/ for the vowel sound. The rhythm of an utterance is affected by stress and also the grouping of thoughts. Properly located pauses are essential in transmitting ideas when speaking. The foreign student concerned with choosing appropriate words while talking may add or improperly locate pauses. The following informal assessment tool may provide helpful information in diagnosing the area of fluency.

Rewrite the following words, eliminating the numbers above them. Instruct the client to orally read them to you. Place a

' over the syllables given primary stress and a " over syllables given secondary stress.

1'-2	1-2'	1'-2-3	1-2'-3	1"-2-3'
carry	receive	instrument	remember	submarine
basket	precede	similar	improvement	overdo
1'-2-3-4	1-2'-3-4	1"-2-3'-4	1"-2-3'-4-5	1-2"-3-4'-5
dangerously	geography	economic	international	communication
accuracy	majority	situation	artificially	misunderstanding

Rewrite the following sentences, eliminating the stress marks indicated. Instruct the client to orally read them. Place a ' over all words stressed by the client.

1. This ring belonged to my mother.

2. Mary is going to put the money in the bank.

3. Who are Bill and Tom taking to the party?

Instruct the client to orally read the following words and phrases. Phonetically transcribe the underlined word to determine if the vowels are obscured or reduced.

1. in a boat	/ə/	5. student	/studənt/
2. big and little	/ən/	6. commandment	/kəmændmənt/
3. two of them	/əv/	7. animal	/ænəməl/
4. go to the store	/tə/	8. repeat	/rəpit/

Instruct the client to first read the following paragraph silently and then orally. Place a / at all places during the verbal reading that the client paused.

The Rainbow Passage

When the sunlight strikes raindrops in the air, they act like a prism and form a rainbow. The rainbow is a division of white light into many beautiful colors. These take the shape of a long round arch, with its path high above, and its two ends apparently beyond the horizon. There is, according to legend, a boiling pot of gold at one end. People look, but no one ever finds it. When a man looks for something beyond his reach, his friends say he is looking for the pot of gold at the end of the rainbow. [Fairbanks, p. 127]

Intonation Assessment

Intonation deals with the pitch changes that occur within an utterance. The intent of a person's statement is very much influenced by the inflectional pattern produced by the speaker. Languages tend to be quite varied in the types of international patterns used. The foreign student may apply his native intonational patterns to English conversation and, consequently, disrupt the listener's ability to comprehend the communicative intent of the message. The diagnostic evaluation should, therefore, include an assessment of intonation patterns such as the following.

Rewrite the following sentences and instruct the client to orally read them. Mark the changes in intonation through the use of a continuous line. The patterns shown are acceptable, but subject to change depending on emphasis.

1. This is the end.
2. What is the answer?
3. Is John sick?
4. We are going either to Florida or Hawaii.
5. Mrs. Smith, here is your coat.
6. You're coming, aren't you?
7. If you bring your ice skates, we can go skating.
8. You're kidding!

Teaching English As a Second Language

Phonological System

If the foreign student is unfamiliar with the production of a large number of English phonemes, it is important to begin instruction with the sound system before attempting word production. This is especially important for the sounds used most frequently in the English language. When reviewing vowel sounds, avoid the use of the long and short vowel classification system as there are many exceptions to this system. Rather, use phonetic symbols or key words to differentiate the various target vowels.

Target Word	Phonetic Symbol	Key Word
man	æ	apple
pin	I	bit
read	i	beet

Core Vocabulary

Since the foreign student has many immediate needs to communicate with the people around him, it is important to begin developing a core vocabulary of words common to his environment. Begin with tangible nouns and verbs that can be easily defined through demonstration and picture. Eventually, this core should include other grammatical forms such as adjectives, adverbs, pronouns, and prepositions. Limit the number of words taught per session so the client will have ample opportunity to retain new words presented to him. It is better to repeatedly present ten to fifteen words rather than to bombard the client with fifty new words. Give a variety of contexts for each vocabulary item as words often change their meaning depending on usage. Note the following example, which takes on a variety of meanings with each new context.

I cut my finger.

Mary cut through Mrs. Kelly's yard.

That's a nasty cut on your arm.

The baby cut two new teeth.

Jack cut class today.

Also include contexts where words are not used, as synonyms are not always interchangeable. For example, one generally *slices* bread rather than *cuts* it.

As vocabulary development continues, train new words through the use of categories. This will help the foreign student to organize the new items. For example, one lesson may concentrate on items found in a drugstore. This would include such words as *ointment, tissues, thermometers,* and *druggist.* Training may be complemented by bringing the actual items into the therapy session.

Another area of vocabulary building that should be emphasized is the use of idioms or slang. Much casual conversation incorporates these forms and, therefore, should be trained to facilitate everyday conversation. Dictionaries of idioms and slang are on the market and may be useful tools in training. Also, the foreign student should be urged to write down any unfamiliar words or phrases heard in conversation.

Morphology

The use of grammatical morphemes is a critical aspect in the development of language in children and, likewise, is very important to the foreign student. Roger Brown (1971) developed a linguistic analysis system to assess spontaneous language samples of children. He found through his research that there was a correlation between the normal child's mean length of utterance (MLU) and the hierarchial order of fourteen grammatical morphemes. Although this analysis system may not be a useful assessment tool for the foreign student, the fourteen grammatical morphemes should be included in the training program. The hierarchy for the training of these structures may be altered to the needs of the foreign student. The fourteen grammatical morphemes include the following:

Present Progressive	Verb + ing
	Going, running
In, On	Used to denote location
	In the box, on the table
Plural	Noun + s (es)
	Boys, girls
Past Irregular	Ran, came
Possessive	Noun + 's
	Mary's, Bill's
Uncontractible Copula	Form of "to be" that does not have the ability to be contracted; Used as main verb; This is Joe.

Articles	A, an, the
Past Regular	Verb + –d + –ed
	Jumped, chased
Third Person Regular	Singular Noun + Verb + s
	Boy eats, cow jumps
Third Person Irregular	Singular noun + does or has
Uncontractible Auxiliary	Form of "to be" that does not have ability to be contracted; Used as a helping verb; The boys are walking. Are they going?
Contractible Copula	Form of "to be" that may be contracted; She is cute. She's cute.
Contractible Auxiliary	Form of "to be" that may be contracted; He is Walking. He's walking.

According to Brown, the developmental order of acquisition of the structures in children is invariant. However, when training these structures with foreign students, the hierarchial order is not as critical. One should note, however, that some of the first grammatical morphemes are prerequisite structures for later morphological forms.

Syntactical Arrangements

Once a core of twenty or more nouns and verbs has been established, begin combining these forms into syntactical arrangements. The following hierarchy is a useful guide in the ordering of the forms to be trained. Sufficiently establish each combination before continuing to the next level by using a variety of words.

S + V V + O	Student eat (s) . Eat supper.
S + V + O	Student eat supper.
S + V + ing + prep + O	Student eating at home.
S + (pl.) + V + ing + prep + O	Students eating at home.

More complex syntactical arrangements should be trained once the hierarchy is completed. Syntax becomes more complex with the addition of such features as articles, adjectives, adverbs, copulas, and auxiliaries.

Articulation

The foreign student often needs to establish new phonemes or variations of similar-sounding phonemes of his native language. This is sometimes a more difficult process than the beginning clinician may anticipate. The articulatory patterning for new phonemes must be incorporated into the already existing patterns of the client's native phonemes, which have become well established from continued use. Consequently, repeated drill is necessary to automatize these articulatory gestures. Each new phoneme should be practiced in a large number of phonemic contexts. The following example demonstrates changing the phonemic context of the target phoneme $/\theta/$ (voiceless *th*).

iθi	Uθi	iθe	Uθe	iθpi	iθfi	iθpe	iθfe
Iθi	oθi	Iθe	oθe	iθbi	iθvi	iθbe	iθve
eθi	ɔθi	eθe	ɔθe	iθti	iθsi	iθte	iθse
εθi	aθi	εθe	aθe	iθdi	iθzi	iθde	iθze
with Pete		with fear		with pay		with fate	
with beans		with Vean		with babies		with vain	
with tea		with seals		with Tate		with saints	
with Dean		with zeal		with Dale		with zany people	

Are you coming with Pete?
I like Mexican dishes with beans.
I eat biscuits with tea.
Mary has a date with Dean.
With fear, Bill approached the stage.
I ate lunch with Dean.
This is the show with seals in it.
The Christians approached with zeal.

New phonemes should be continuously drilled until they become automatic. The clinician may wish to send home tape-recorded samples of the target phoneme so the foreign student has a model to match when practicing. Auditory discrimination tasks involving the target phoneme and commonly substituted sounds may also provide additional feedback to the client.

Intonation

Intonation may well be one of the major factors affecting the foreign students "accent." The English language has much variability in its intonation patterns, and considerable meaning is derived from the type of pitch change used. Intonation in some foreign languages is not as critical a feature as it is in English, and therefore, it may be a difficult characteristic for a foreign speaker to incorporate into a second language. Some languages, on the other hand, have a highly refined intonation system, which may cause some interference when a new language is attempted.

The foreign student should practice using a variety of English intonation patterns. When training these patterns, it is not necessary for the student to match the clinician's pitch level, but rather that his voice indicates a pitch change in the proper direction. The following are examples of intonation patterns common to the English language as defined by Prator (1951). Note that a gliding pattern is used if the last sentence stress comes on the last syllable of the sentence.

1. Rising-falling. This type of intonation is generally used in declarative sentences, commands, and questions using interrogative pronouns.

DECLARATIVE SENTENCES

a. The sky is blue.

b. Mary looks sad.

c. This is my grandson.

d. I bought a new bicycle.

COMMANDS

a. Shut the door.

b. Untie Joe's shoe.

c. Open the cupboard.

d. Eat all of your potatoes.

QUESTIONS WITH INTERROGATIVE PRONOUNS

a. What color is his hair?

b. Why are you here?

c. Where did you put the pencil?

d. How are you feeling?

2. Rising.   This type of pitch variation is generally used with questions not beginning with interrogative pronouns.   Any statement may be changed to a question by simply using this intona-

QUESTIONS WITHOUT INTERROGATIVE PRONOUNS

a. Is this you friend?   c. Are you going to the store?

b. Do you have a piece of candy?   d. Will you buy me some licorice?

STATEMENTS CHANGED TO QUESTIONS

a. He bought a new car?   c. You are going to the dentist's?

b. She is leaving for Alaska?   d. You like spinach?

DIRECT ADDRESS

a. Mrs. Jones, it's so good to meet you.

b. I'm happy to see you, old buddy.

c. Bring me the paper, Susan.

d. Uncle Joe, I'm looking forward to your visit.

tion pattern.   Words of direct address use a similar rising pattern.

3. Combination Rising and Rising-Falling.   All members of a series of words connected by *and* or *or* use a rising pattern except the last member, which uses a rising-falling pattern.

a. I ate popcorn, pizza, and a hotdog.

b. I bought shoes, a hat, and an umbrella.

c. Are you going to Hawaii or Florida?

d. Shall we go to the museum, the fair, or the theater?

4. Rising-Falling to Normal Pitch.   This type of intonation occurs at the end of a thought group, which indicates that additional information will follow.

a. I finished the dishes, so I will go outside.

b. Mary is a good seamstress, but sometimes she cuts corners.

c. I'd like to go to the circus, but I think I'd better stay here.

d. If you give me a mop, I'll clean up the floor.

5. Tag-On Questions.   Intonation varies with this type of structure between rising-falling and rising patterns.   A rising-falling

pattern indicates that the speaker does not expect a response whereas the rising pattern does expect the listener to respond.

a. You're going to the game, aren't you? (expects a response)
b. You're going to the game, aren't you? (no response)
c. It's a nice day, isn't it? (expects response)
d. It's a nice day, isn't it? (no response)

6. Exceptions. Exceptions to the above rules may exist when a speaker wishes to draw special attention to a certain portion of the sentence. Note how the following statements vary in their intonation depending on the emphasis given to the sentence. The foreign student should practice changing his intonation according to the questions the clinician asks.

a. Who gave the book?   The boy gave the book to his father.
b. What did the boy give?   The boy gave the book to his father.
c. To whom did the boy give the book? The boy gave the book to his father.
d. Whose father was it?   The boy gave the book to his father.

A useful tool in training intonation outside the therapy session is through the use of tape-recorded samples. The clinician should tape a variety of patterns so the client may have a model to copy. It is this author's experience that foreign students often lack good English models as their circle of friends tends to be speakers of their native tongue or family members.

Fluency

With each new vocabulary word trained, the accent or stress within the word should also be emphasized. The client should be instructed that stress is the result of increased loudness and an elevated pitch level. Additional emphasis is placed on the stressed syllable by reducing the vowel sound in the unstressed syllable to a /ə/ or /I/. Note the following examples, which demonstrate stress within words.

jacket   /dʒǽkət/

robin   /rάbən/

carpet	/kárpət/
about	/əbaʊ́t/
remember	/rɪmɛ́mbɚ/

Stress within sentences should also be practiced. Generally, content words, or words carrying meaning in and of themselves, are stressed within a sentence. Function words, those words conveying little meaning, are unstressed. Content words involve such grammatical classes as nouns, verbs, adjectives, and adverbs. Function words include articles, prepositions, and conjunctions. The following sentences have the content words marked.

1. The óld mán wálked across the strèet.
2. Máry boúght a néw dréss.
3. Jóe áte síx páncakes.
4. Bíll and Ríck pláy sóftball óften.
5. The bóy sáng a beaútiful sóng.

Stress within words and sentences is subject to change depending on the intent of the speaker. However, it is better for the foreign student to first learn the general rule before incorporating the exceptions into the training program.

A third area influencing the fluency of speech is proper location of pauses within thought groups. Location of pauses is generally dependent upon the speaker; however, some general rules do apply. For example, pauses between thought groups occur at the end of a statement and never occur between related words such as an adjective and a noun. Improper placement of pauses frequently disrupts the communicative intent of the message and becomes difficult for the listener to understand.

An initial step in training a foreign student to speak in thought groups is to mark a passage with slashes, indicating pauses. The client should orally read the passage until the pauses become natural. The following is an example of such a passage.

I go fishing up in Maine every summer./ Personally/I am very fond of strawberries and cream;/but I find that for some strange reason/fish prefer worms./ So/when I go fishing, /I don't think about what I want./ I think about what they want./ I don't bait the hook with strawberries and cream./ Rather,/ I dangle a worm or a grasshopper in front of the fish and say:/ "Wouldn't you like to have that?"/

from *How to Win Friends and Influence People*
by Dale Carnegie

Eventually, the client himself should be instructed to mark the passages with slashes before orally reading them. Once this task becomes easy for the client, delete the slashes completely and have the client simply read passages aloud. Role-playing situations may be helpful techniques in establishing carryover from the written prose to conversation.

Summary

This chapter has suggested that the training of English as a second language is not a unique instructional program but rather encompasses all the major aspects of speech and language remediation. The major variation from other therapy populations that does occur from the fact that the foreign student has already established a native language. Consequently, the first language may at times interfere with second language learning and other times facilitate it.

A thorough diagnostic workup should begin the training program so the client's English performance level may be determined. Once this level is derived, training should begin at a level where some success in the usage of English is achieved. Continual, drill-oriented activities are necessary so English usage becomes automatic. Good English-speaking models are also critical aspects of the training program.

References

Ammons, R. and Ammons, H.: Full-Range Picture Vocabulary Test. Missoula, Montana: Psychological Test Specialists, 1958.

Brown, R.: *A First Language*. Cambridge, Mass.: Harvard University Press, 1973.

Carnegie, D.: *How to Win Friends and Influence People*. New York: Simon and Schuster, 1964.

Carrow, E.: Test for Auditory Comprehension of Language (5th ed.). Austin, Texas: Learning Concepts, 1974.

Dunn, L. Peabody Picture Vocabulary Test. Minneapolis: American Guidance Service, Inc., 1965.

Fairbanks, G. *Voice and Articulation Book* (2nd ed). New York: Harper and Row, 1960.

Foster, R., Giddan, J., and Stark, J.: ACLC: Assessment of Children's Language Comprehension. Palo Alto, Calif.: Consulting Psychologists Press, 1969.

Kirk, S., McCarthy, J., and Kirk, W.: The Illinois Test of Psycholinguistic Abilities (Rev. ed.). Urbana: University of Illinois Press, 1968.

Prator, C.: *Manual of American English Pronunciation* (Rev. Ed.). New York: Holt, Rinehart and Winston, 1957.

Chapter 5

ARTICULATION

SR. MARIE KOPIN

OVERVIEW

ARTICULATION remediation programs can be one of the more challenging aspects of the clinical case load of any speech pathologist. Problems can range from a single consistent sound error to complex involvements of multi-handicapped individuals who lack the complete motor and/or neurological basis to develop normal speech articulation skills. Articulation disorders can often be combined with problems in developmental language handicaps, neurological deficits, cultural differences, and mental handicaps.

Speech pathologists work with many other professionals. This is a comforting thought, and should not be forgotten. The clinician can rely on others to assist with the treatment of speech problems. Any individual having contact with a communicatively handicapped person has potential to assist or hinder progress in speech. The clinician who can harness the potential teaching talents of persons in a client's environs can often double efforts. A "team" effort of parents, teachers, hospital staff, peers, and others can be enriching to all concerned. Knowledge of theories of articulation disorders is essential, but practical applications must be made in a client's total surroundings. A letter, as illustrated in Figure 5-1, sent to staff may help clarify the clinician's position.

Various settings for clinical work also offer unique challenges as does keeping up with the progress of scientific research and cultural change. The clinical work in schools is demanding and

THE ROLE OF SPEECH THERAPIST

It is essential that the speech therapist evaluate the severity of every speech problem that is referred to her. Not every child with poor speech is a candidate for speech therapy. It is necessary to determine whether a child's speech needs can be met through regular attention given to speech development by the classroom teacher or whether he requires more specialized attention.

Every child referred to the therapist for evaluation is categorized as having a mild, moderate, or severe defect of phonation, language structure, rhythm, or misarticulations of sounds. According to P.L. 94-142, the speech therapist is given the responsibility for determining which children are in need of speech rehabilitation.

One of the prime objectives of a therapist is to create the sort of environment in which his pupils can develop their own potentialities to the greatest extent possible. Every child must do his own changing, his own learning, rather than having it done for him. It must be remembered, however, that these changes may take a long time to occur. Many months, or sometimes even several years of constant therapy are necessary for a child to overcome a speech defect.

Changes within the child mean changes in deeper-lying attitudes, perceptions, needs, values, and goals, which make it possible for him to change his behavior. Encouragement and support of the family, teacher, and classmates are the important factors in determining how soon the correct speech pattern will replace the old, incorrect one in the child's everyday speech.

The following criteria are necessary for the cooperation of the regular teaching staff of the school:

a. It is important that the speech therapist see the students at work in their regular classrooms; this is done with the approval of the principal.

b. The regular teacher can be of assistance to the therapist in creating a proper attitude on the part of the child toward the speech assignments by referring to them as a part of his school work. This will be a help to the boys and girls in their conduct through the halls to and from speech class.

c. The speech therapist may have suggestions for the regular classroom teacher to assist the speech defective child in overcoming his problem.

Figure 5-1. Letter to staff. From Speech Therapy Department, Board of Education, Cleveland, Ohio. Reprinted by Permission.

includes the coordination of work with other professionals and with parents, and keeping up on new laws about mandatory aid to the handicapped. There are many opportunities to extend programs by training teachers, parents, and volunteers to assist; thus, managerial skills are also necessary. One of the advantages of working in a school is that there can be years of long-term contact with the same client.

The hospital setting offers the speech clinician the challenge of being a member of a highly trained team including members of the medical profession. There is the daily excitement of new clientele with severe disabilities. Articulation therapy in this setting often includes the more severe, short-term client of pre-school or post-school age.

WHAT IS AN ARTICULATION DISORDER?

Many authors have given overview descriptions of articulation problems, from any difficulty an individual has when he uses the speech sounds of the language spoken around him, to the classic definition of Van Riper (1937), which is still one of the most commonly used. Van Riper states that a speech disorder (1) draws attention to itself, (2) interferes with communication, and (3) disturbs the communicator.

If some phase of articulation is disturbing to the speaker and/ or listener(s), a problem does indeed exist. Examples include the small child who knows others do not understand him, the highly intelligent foreign visitor who wishes s/he could not be detected by his/her pronunciation, or the person who wishes to remove more subtle traces of some regional dialect.

Articulation disorders should be viewed as more than an inability to produce a particular sound (Winitz, 1977). McReynolds and Huston (1971) have shown that functional articulation errors do not necessarily reflect inabilities in production alone. Deficiencies in the learning experience that may not be directly evident are also involved. Some audiologists, for instance, claim that even a short-term, mild loss at a critical stage of development can affect learning.

ARTICULATION THERAPY, THE BASIC WORK
OF THE SPEECH PATHOLOGIST

Children with articulation problems usually constitute the majority of the case load of most speech pathologists, especially in school settings. The beginner is often anxious to begin drill and work on "sounds" right away; however, there are important questions to be asked at the initiation of therapy. How does one deal successfully with the *person* who has the disorder; will this *client* become better as a person and more proficient in total communication skills as a result of contacts with the speech pathologist; how does the disorder affect her/his life now and in the future; how can this future be improved with the assistance of the speech clinician?

FIFTY YEARS OF PROGRESS IN A CHANGING TIME

Methods in articulation therapy have been developing over the past fifty years. In the beginning days of speech programs in schools, clinicians found dozens of children with articulation disorders in every grade. Pupils who were older took longer to correct. Large groups of clients, sometimes fifteen, were taken for half-hour periods. Today's work is much different. The incidence of articulation problems in older pupils has decreased in school districts where programs have existed for ten or more years. The only high school students needing work today are those in unserved schools; those who moved in from unserved schools; those who "like" their difficulties; and those with hearing, motor, mental retardation, or physical handicaps, which have made years of therapy necessary.

Modern research has also revealed much more about the normal sequence of speech and language acquisition (Winitz, 1969, 1975; Brown, 1973) and about the nature of learning. Various programs and methods have been developed to fit the needs of a variety of clients and clinicians in every setting. Much research has endeavored to answer the question, How does the client learn most effectively?; but there is little research on what makes a good clinician (Mowrer, 1969).

Since the number of age ten and above clients with single and double sound problems has decreased in the last fifteen years, the clinician often works with the more challenging very young or older clients. More stress is placed on the stimulation and development of skills of the preschool client. The term *speech correction* may be outdated because more and more work is being done to develop accurate speech rather than "correct" long-standing habitual sound distortions, omissions, and substitutions.

There are many methods and techniques of articulation remediation in several "classic" reference texts; recommended references include Sommers and Kane (1974), Eisenson and Ogilvie (1977), Powers (1971), Van Riper (1972, 1978).

In the beginning days of clinical work, much emphasis was placed upon direct drill and individual work with clients (Van Riper, 1972). Some clinicians relied on manipulation of mouths, and crude appliances were used to position the articulators. Strong sound-stimulation techniques recommended by Travis (1931) and Van Riper (1937) promoted auditory training. Edna Hill Young carried stimulation techniques further with "moto-kinesthetic" approaches (1938). All of these approaches usually combined individual therapy with solid drill approaches.

In 1947, Backus and Dunn began to promote use of therapy groups to make use of conversational techniques. Ollie Backus developed this further and eventually joined forces with Jane Beasley, stressing use of "carrier phrases" in a more natural conversational setting for children as opposed to the direct drill used by many before them. Their book, *Speech Therapy with Children* (1958), outlines the method.

Clinicians began adopting and developing new objective techniques and systems for articulation analysis and remediation. The development of linguistic studies has stimulated top clinicians, including Eugene MacDonald and Janis Costello, to develop their "Sensorimotor" and "Distinctive Features" approaches redefining more intimate sound relationships. Advanced acoustic and visual machines present more challenges as do computerized systems for recording data and retrieving information. Emphasis is also continually shifting towards development of speech in the young, preventive therapy, work with the retarded, and the Senior Citizen. Who knows what the future holds?

CLASSIC TECHNIQUES AND APPROACHES

The following list includes some classic techniques and approaches that are well accepted in many clinical settings:

1. *Traditional Therapy.* This is a term usually referring to therapy with groups of clients using approaches originally outlined by Backus and Beasly (1951) and the early editions of Van Riper's books. Specific terms connected with Traditional Therapy include *phonetic placement, key word, stimulation, auditory training, negative practice,* and *carrier phrase.*

2. PHONETIC PLACEMENT (Scripture, 1927; Nemoy and Davis, 1937; Van Riper, 1972. The clinician tells the client specifically how to place the articulators to produce a given sound (target sound). Pictures, models, and charts may be used to visually demonstrate correct placement, e.g. "Form-a-sound" cards, dental plaster cast teeth, drawings and illustrations in books.

3. *Key Word* (Van Riper, 1972). This term simply means the client is given a common word containing his/her target sound to remember. Hopefully, s/he remembers to say the given word correctly during the day as well as correct usage in various contexts in speech class. *Key Word* is a term that has been in use many years.

4. *Stimulus method* (Van Riper, 1972) Strong stimulation using syllables containing the target sound is advised. The clinician literally floods the client with stimulation such as, "See-Saw-Say-So-Sue; again, See, saw, say, so, sue; again, See-saw-say-so-sue; now say, So!" This type of exercise is drilled and repeated during remediation sessions.

5. *Stimulation* (Van Riper, 1972). The client is presented with a strong, clear, and appropriate model of the target sound by the clinician and is motivated to reproduce it.

6. *Negative Practice* (Van Riper, 1972) Negative practice refers to the client producing the speech error purposely to study the feel and sound of the old and new articulation pattern of a target sound.

7. *Motokinesthetic* (Young and Stichfield-Hawk, 1955; and

Tjomsland, 1968) . The client's mouth is manipulated by the clinician, who touches certain speech-related tissues to suggest movement. The client is taught to feel the inner movements of the articulators and to respond with a new-found kinesthetic awareness.

8. *Group therapy Carrier Phrase* (Backus and Beasley, 1951). The use of the *carrier phrase* in a natural conversational setting was developed by Backus and Beasley. This was a word or phrase (commonly used) that contained the target sound, e.g. target sound of /s/. For example, "May I please take a piece"; "Yes, you may." This phrase idea was to be used in a group as the clients interacted with each other using objects or real-life activities.

9. *Scanning and Monitoring* (Van Riper and Irwin, 1958) A client can be trained to "scan" and "inspect" the variety of sounds his articulators produce. S/he is encouraged by the therapist to develop a system of self-monitoring and awareness of production of the correct target sound. Auditory training and feedback are emphasized. Kinesthetic and tactile feedback are also employed.

10. *Feedback Theory* (Mysak, 1971) . This idea emphasizes the importance of feedback during interaction with a client. Both feedback from the clinician and developing feedback systems in the client are important. This is a modern version of Van Riper and Irwin's "Scanning and Monitoring" (1958) .

11. *Sensorimotor Skills and Sounds in Relationships* (McDonald, 1964) . The use of awareness of senses and relationships of a target sound to other sounds in varying contexts is stressed. Drill on the /s/ would include mastery of many different contexts of vowels and consonants in combination with the /s/ sound.

12. *Behavior Modification Techniques* (Baker and Ryan, 1971; Mowrer, 1975; Keller, 1954; Psaltis and Spalatto, 1973). This approach emphasizes shaping the client's behavior by means of reinforcement of actions. It is a technique used by all good teachers, but new terminology and thorough

research have clarified systematic ways to use rewards for increasing good and appropriate speech behaviors.

13. *Programmed Instructional Approaches* (Baker and Ryan, 1971; Mowrer, 1968; 1978; Psaltis and Spallato, 1973). Janis Costello (1977) gives a good overview of these types of approaches. They all have one thing in common, a complete manual of systematic material on remediation of a particular sound with complete, step-by-step instructions for the clinician and client. Both teaching and learning behaviors are specified *a priori*. The things needed most are a sensitive ear, immediate and accurate feedback, and a willingness to depart from a structured lesson to adapt to individual needs of clients.

14. *Paired Stimulus* (Irwin, 1971; Irwin and Weston, 1971; Weston and Irwin, 1973). This unique technique uses a combination of the known and unknown. A word easily produced is paired with ten or more phonetically similar words containing the target sound. Behavior modification techniques are used to set up a reinforcement schedule as the client practices. The words are always paired, the known with the unknown.

15. *Precision Skills* (Mowrer, 1971; Williams, 1973; Toohey, 1975; Waters, 1957). This refers to the use of behavior modification techniques and precise, immediate clinician feedback to each response of the client. The speech lesson is skillfully geared at the client's level so that no more than one error occurs in four responses. Then precise and accurate feedback is given for each response; these responses are counted and recorded by the clinician and client so an accurate count of progress is obtained. Waters (1975) suggests that this therapy approach consists of gathering and analyzing baseline data, determining behavior objectives, arranging antecedent and consequent events to insure a high total-response rate and a low error-response rate, recording responses, graphing progress, and setting criteria for each learned behavior. The interplay of these components is important. The process is more than a step-by-step procedure because manipulation of various compon-

ents is controlled by clinical judgements. This procedure can be applied to group work as well as individuals.

16. *Reading and Speech Therapy.* Combining reading at various levels with speech lessons can achieve desirable results. The printed word containing target sounds is a visual reminder of the presence of a particular sound. The client is also apt to remember to use a target sound better during language arts classes and/or other reading times. Skills in reading may also be improved as word attack skills are directly related to auditory discrimination and memory skills.

17. *Distinctive Features* (Costello, 1975; Costello and Onstine, 1976; McReynolds and Engmann, 1975; McReynolds and Bennett, 1972; and Pollack and Rees, 1972). This term, which is relatively recent in the literature of speech pathology, refers to a complete analysis of all the acoustic features of a sound relating these characteristics to sounds containing similar features. Thus, an entire family of related sounds may be selected for target sound work, all at the same time.

SPEECH SCREENING

The quick speech screening is a valuable and necessary device for a speech clinician who must identify speech-impaired clients among large groups of people. This is especially true in the school setting. There are a number of tasks to be completed to ensure a fast and thorough job that satisfies everyone involved:

1. Professionals involved with the groups should be asked for referrals (see Fig. 5-2). These professionals can be trained at staffings or at other meetings before the screening program begins. Training can include a talk and demonstration of various types of speech problems and establishment of a comfortable rapport with the speech pathologist. They should be made aware of the possible scope of a total speech program, including the type of services children can receive and consultative help for parents and professionals. A simple referral form may be used (see Fig. 5-3), or the clinician could be given names of individuals to check more

Dear Teacher:

We are at present in the process of forming new speech classes for the school year. At this time, it will be necessary to conduct speech screening tests. We have the files of students in your school who have previously attended speech class, and all of these students will be notified and retested. As a teacher, you may have noticed children in your classroom who do not speak plainly. This can result from problems of (1) Articulation, (2) Rhythm, or (3) Voice.

If a child does not speak clearly, especially after six or seven years of age, he probably has an articulatory problem. Under this classification will be found (1) Substitutions (wed instead of red), (2) Omissions (kool instead of school), (3) Insertions (stun instead of sun), and (4) Distortions. The lisper falls within this group. His [s], [z], and sometimes [sh] and [ch] may be affected. For example, the tongue protrudes between the teeth, causing the child to say "thee" instead of "see." Difficulty with [r] (run) and [l] (let) are often other common articulatory problems.

Stuttering and cluttering are both classified as problems of rhythm. Stuttering is an interruption of the normal rhythm of speech. It is characterized by relatively effortless repetitions of sounds and prolongations of words and syllables, or by complete blocks when speech is attempted. Often, the stuttering spasm is accompanied by blinking of eyes, sniffs, and by twitching of facial, shoulder, and hand muscles. It is recognized that the severity of the stuttering block will depend upon the individual and the situation, so a great deal can be done toward helping the stutterer by making his surroundings as calm as possible.

Cluttering is produced by too rapid a rate of speech, characterized by slurred and omitted syllables and consonants, improper phrasing, and speech sounds distorted by speed.

Voice problems are not prevalent in children, but they do occur occasionally. They are classified as problems of pitch (too high or too low), quality (too husky, too breathy, too nasal or denasal), volume (too soft or too loud), and monotonous inflection. There is an especially great range of normal performance in relation to voice.

Please watch for the child with indications of any of these defects and immediately refer him to the speech therapist. In this way we can organize the classes within the next few weeks and permit any child who needs assistance to obtain it as soon as possible and thus benefit most from speech class.

In the spaces below, please write the names of any students in your room who, you feel, would benefit from speech class. If you are uncertain of whether a child has a speech difficulty, list his name anyway. For each child please add a brief statement of what the problem seems to be. You may return this form to the office mailbox. As soon as the final speech class schedule is formed, I will send a copy to you.

Thank you very much for your cooperation in this matter. If at any time during the school year you feel another child would benefit from speech correction, please notify me. We will try to place the child in class, if possible.

Sincerely,

Speech Therapist

_____

_____

_____

_____

_____

_____

Figure 5-2. Referral letter to teachers. From Speech Therapy Department, Board of Education, Cleveland, Ohio. Reprinted by permission.

carefully as screening progresses. A sheet describing possible articulation errors is also helpful to staff (see Fig. 5-4).

2. The actual screening process should be scheduled well enough in advance so all are prepared and the speech clinician is welcomed into the classroom or group. A simple introduction of the speech pathologist is in order with a short explanation made that everyone will be speaking to her/him in turn. Clients should be put in groups of three to five persons, who are then directed to go, one group at a time, wherever the clinician is situated (corner of the room, hall, special room in the building, office etc.). The area should be as quiet as possible. When one person is finished, s/he goes at once to get the next small group; no time is to be lost.

3. The listening ability of the clinician is *critical*. The clinician proceeds to ask the client(s) to count, name colors, recite the alphabet, and name some objects, e.g. "chair,

```
Date:_____

To:  Teachers at_____School.

Re:  Speech, Language, and Hearing Program

We are beginning a new semester of school. Please fill out the following in
regards to children you would like referred for speech, language, and/or
hearing services this semester. Place the bottom half of this sheet in the
principal's office by_____

Thanks for cooperating,


_____
Speech Clinician


                                    tear here
-----------------------------------------------------------------------------

Teacher's name_____ room number_____

Grade_____

I would like these students checked for speech, language, and/or hearing.

Name                              Problem
```

Figure 5-3. Referral form. From Speech Therapy Department, Board of Education, Cleveland, Ohio. Reprinted by permission.

Enunciation	This word describes "running speech" instead of a single word.

Omission of letters — Examples:

Wrong	Correct
wanna	want to
canchoo	can't you
jus	just

Slur — Words jumbled together — Examples:

Wrong	Correct
Jeet yet?	did you eat yet?
No, Joo?	No, did you?
Wyen-cheet-wious?	Why don't you eat with us?

Pronunciation	This word refers to the use of the single word and its use of sound when used separately by itself. Examples:

Wrong	Correct
dees and dose	these and those
tanks	thanks
runnin	running
(short *i* for short *e* in — git	get

Omission — Leaving out letters. Examples:

Wrong	Correct
wan	want
des	desk
jus	just

Sound reversals — Here the letters are not in their proper place. Examples:

Wrong	Correct
aks	ask
hunderd	hundred

Addition — Extra letters are put in. Examples:

Wrong	Correct
oncet	once
acrosst	across
twicet	twice

Stress — This means putting the accent in the right place.

Wrong	Correct
po'lice	police'

Figure 5-4. Articulation errors. From Speech Therapy Department, Board of Education, Cleveland, Ohio. Reprinted by permission.

thumb, face, cheeks, shoe, dress, leg." These one-word responses should be words that contain sounds commonly misarticulated. If anything is suspected, the clinician may find a memorized list of sentences with major speech sounds helpful; the client is asked to repeat the sentences after the tester. The list (Fig. 5-5) by Harlan Bloomer is a good one, as is the sentence articulation test in the Fisher-Logeman Test. Clients aged ten and older may be asked to read from an easy book. Others may be asked to recite commonly memorized materials (scout pledge, the Pledge of Allegiance, nursery rhymes). The Triota Word Test by Irwin

1. Sassy mice race across the ice.
   Zippers are easy to close.
2. Why whisper everywhere?
   We will win anyway.
3. Think nothing but the truth.
   This leather is smooth.
4. Shaving lotion will splash.
   Measure the position of the garage.
5. Choose a pitcher to match.
   John put a pigeon in the cage.
6. Find the office knife.
   Violets cover the grove.
7. Lend me a ruler and pencil.
   Mama made some lemon jam.
8. Wrap the carrots with paper.
   New pennies shine.
9. Your onions are yellow.
   Bring the singer along.
10. Tie a better knot.
    Daddy nodded his head.
11. Keep the pocket book.
    Go get a bigger egg.
12. Papa put paper in the pipe.
    Buy baby a bib.
13. He hit his hand anyhow.

1. Ho't
2. Ha't
3. He'ck
4. Hay'
5. Hi't
6. He'
7. Haw'k
8. Hut'
9. Her'
10. Hoe'
11. Hoo'k
12. Who'
13. High'
14. How'
15. Hoi'st
16. Hue'

Figure 5-5. Bloomer Sentence Articulation Test. From Harlan Bloomer, University of Michigan Speech Clinic. Reprinted by permission.

(1972) is also convenient (see Figure 5-6) . If suspicions are confirmed, then the name of the client can be written on a 3 by 5 inch index card and coded as to type of difficulty, severity, age, and class. The client is then sent back to the room, the teacher or monitor informed after all the screenings, and the client then scheduled for a more lengthy diagnosis at a later time. Use of the 3 by 5 inch cards also makes scheduling convenient later. These cards can be coded with colors and numbers.

4. Feedback to the teacher or other professional in charge of the group is extremely important at this time. They will have questions and will provide comments and insights as well as assisting in follow-through scheduling and treatment.

TRIOTA TEN WORD TEST

Scoring instructions: For omission, distortion, or addition error, place code number. in the space to the right of the diagonal line. For substitution, enter the phonetic symbol for the sound substituted. Leave the space to the right of the diagonal blank if the phoneme is articulated socially acceptably.

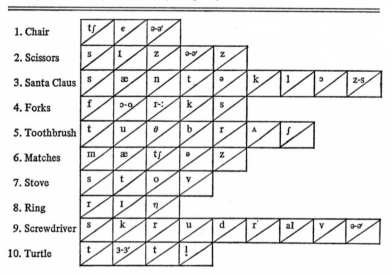

Figure 5-6. Triota Word Test. From "The Triota: A Computerized Battery" by J. Irwin, *Acta Symbolica, 3*:26-38, 1972.

5. Making an overall report of screening results to be given to all professional staff and administrators involved is very important. A specific listing of clients with a brief indication of their problems (type and severity) will alert all the staff as to their needs as well as impress administrators with the total needs for speech, language, and hearing therapy within their schools. A good screening summary could result in hiring of additional staff and/or in better scheduling and total program planning.

6. How often should screenings be done? Each situation should be studied as to its needs. A new clinician may wish to do a total program screening as an important get acquainted procedure. An administrator may also request one for total planning needs. The clinician may screen vital age groups regularly every year as well as certain other types of children. A suggested list of yearly screenings for the school setting follows:

    1. All preschoolers.

    2. All kindergarteners and first graders.

    3. All third or fourth graders.

    4. The top grade level in any building.

    5. Senior High classes (12th grade).

    6. All those who previously had speech within 3 years of dismissal time.

    7. All teacher referrals.

    8. All those in special classes and/or resource center programs.

    9. Children on a waiting list.

Screenings can be done at the beginning or at the end of the school year, or any time the children need to be surveyed. Volunteers and/or teacher aides can be helpful to assist. In the Cleveland, Ohio Public Schools an entire building of 500 to 1000 pupils is often screened in a day with the help of extra therapists on their coordination time. One class of twenty-five pupils need not take more than twenty minutes.

ACCEPTING A CLIENT

What are the criteria for accepting a client for enrollment in a speech program? Many factors need to be considered, and there is no easy formula.

Consideration should first of all be made of the total person's needs and his/her willingness (or parent's willingness) to accept help. The cooperation and desire of older clients, age ten and over, is especially important. It is the speech clinician's job to interview, study, and evaluate the client, his/her needs, and possibilities for enrollment. The reason for referral should be carefully noted as should the comments and reasons given by the referral source whether it be parents, peers, family, other professionals, or another speech pathologist. The number, scope, type, and range of sound errors, intelligibility of connected speech, and accompanying sensory and language deficits should be considered.

The diadochokinetic rate of production of /p-t-k/ sequencing abilities should also be checked. Bloomquist (1950), Maxwell (1953), and Irwin and Becklund (1953) have established age norms for speech-motor movements. The idea is that, if the client can sequence p-t-k easily (at least 4 or 5 per second), the prognosis for correction of error sounds is very good. Clients who cannot sequence these three sounds easily are candidates for high priority on a case load.

Length of treatment should be estimated and the client, responsible professional, and/or parents informed at the onset. This is the time to begin to formulate a well-designed program of treatment, which must be made known to all involved.

There has been some recent rethinking and study of the priorities of selection of clients of school age (Hatten and Laroque, 1972). The following hierarchy for selection is recommended:

1. *First* take any pupils of intermediate grade level or older, especially in previously unserved settings.
2. *Second,* clients of preschool, first grade, and kindergarten ages with multiple articulation problems, lateral lisps, and/ or accompanying organic handicaps and learning disabilities should be taken. Both parents and clients of this age are eager and easily trained. A program using consultation

with willing parents and older siblings can be invaluable even if the children are only occasionally seen by the speech clinician.

3. *Third,* clients from grades two and three with single and/or double sound substitutions should be considered last.

4. *Fourth,* it is expected, too, that the clinician will keep a list of clients at carryover stages. These children should be seen monthly or checked only on occasion.

This scheme, admittedly, contradicts the traditional notion of not taking kindergarten or first grade clients but has been tried with success in many schools in Ohio and Michigan. More research and study are indicated here.

GETTING THE CASE HISTORY

If no previous records are available, the clinician must begin to gather information in a usable form. Parents/Guardians can be given forms to fill out and return. This information can then be summarized and used as a basis for a parent meeting. The Cleveland Public Schools use a "clinician designed" pocket folder form for diagnostic and case history notes and recording progress (Fig. 5-7). Important facts relating to birth problems, age of speaking, diseases, injuries, ear infections, emotional traits, age and number of siblings and adults in the home, history of family speech problems, and home conditions should be noted.

INFORMING THE PARENTS

Parents should be informed about their child and the problem at all times. The first contact is especially important. The new federal laws mandating special education services are to be followed in arranging a planning meeting with parents and other school personnel for the purpose of enrolling a child in speech rehabilitation in the school setting. Children may be referred from the school setting to a variety of agencies. A sample letter to parents about an initial meeting and initial enrollment in speech is found in Figure 5-8.

SPEECH RECORD – DEPARTMENT OF SPEECH THERAPY – CLEVELAND PUBLIC SCHOOLS

AGE																
GRADE																
ROOM NO.																

LAST NAME FIRST MIDDLE

ADDRESS BIRTHDATE TEL. NO.

ADDRESS | ADDRESS

ADDRESS | ADDRESS

RECORD OF PREVIOUS SPEECH THERAPY

School	Date Begun	Date Ended	Cause of Termination	Speech Therapist

AUDIOLOGICAL EVALUATIONS

Date	Type	Air Cond. R	Air Cond. L	Bone Cond. R	Bone Cond. L	Recommendations

INTELLECTUAL AND OTHER EVALUATIONS

Date	Test	Agency	CA	MA	IQ

PROFESSIONAL CONTACTS (NON-PUBLIC SCHOOL)

Date	Agency or Person	Results or Recommendations

SPEECH EXAMINATION AND EVALUATION

GENERAL OBSERVATIONS OF SPEECH	LATERALITY	ARTICULATION	PHONETIC CHECK LIST	I	M	F	Corr.
Fluency		Functional					
Language Level	HEARING LOSS SYMPTOMS	Organic					
	Speech	Oral Inactivity	s				
Grammar, Pronunciation	Voice		z				
Foreign Accent, Dialect	Behavior	Oral Inaccuracy	th				
Visible Aspects			th̲				
	LANGUAGE		ng				
Intelligibility	Receptive	Lisp (Type)	r				
			y				
ORGANIC DEVIATIONS	Expressive	Multiple Artic.	h				
Structure			wh				
Oral Cavity	VOICE		l				
Palate	Pitch	Ability to Imitate Sounds	j				
Tonsils, Adenoids	Loudness		ch				
Tongue	Quality		sh				
Teeth	Rate	Vowels	k				
Jaws	Rhythm		q				
Lips	Hypernasality		f				
Nose		Consonant Blends	v				
Miscellaneous	STUTTERING		Others				
MUSCULAR COORDINATION		EVALUATION					
Speech Mechanism							
General		PROGNOSIS					

CASE HISTORY DATE TAKEN

A. FAMILY

	SIBLINGS (INDICATE CASE'S POSITION WITH ARROW)
FATHER Nationality	Name Age Speech Other
Occupation	1.
Speech	2.
Other	3.
MOTHER Nationality	4.
Occupation	5.
Speech	
Other	

HOME CONDITIONS

B. CHILD

DEVELOPMENT: AGE OF WALKING Words Sentences

Birth Dental History Habits

HEALTH: DISEASES

Operations Accidents

Defects, Problems Present Health

Educational and Achievement Factors

Personality, Behavior, Social Adjustment

SPEECH PROBLEM: ONSET

Course of Development

Family Reactions

Figure 5-7. Case history. From Speech Therapy Department, Board of Education, Cleveland, Ohio. Reprinted by permission.

PREPARING FOR THE FIRST MEETING WITH A CLIENT

The initial meeting with the client can set the tone for the entire therapy program. The clinician is wise to prepare beforehand by reviewing the case in a variety of ways:

1. Speaking with the referral source(s);
2. Referring to notes on screening and/or brief interviews before therapy is formally initiated;
3. Studying professional records, the case history, school reports, and previous diagnoses by various disciplines;
4. Reviewing the type of articulation problem and selecting test material to assist in choosing the therapy target sound(s) and to establish a baseline;
5. Checking the reason for referral;
6. Deciding whether to use group or individualized therapy as the most efficient and beneficial means of a program for the clients' needs and means;
7. Checking to see if a basic general articulation test has been

Dear Parents:

The federal government has implemented a new Mandatory Education Act, P.L. 94-142. This law states that all speech and language pathologists must obtain written permission from parents prior to screening and/or evaluating their children. The law also requires Individual Educational Planning (IEP) meetings with each parent prior to accepting their child into therapy. Specific objectives, outlining methods, materials, and prognosis, must be developed for each child and presented to the parents for their consent.

I must meet with you prior to October 1,   in order to enroll your child in the speech therapy program. If I do not meet with you and receive your written consent, your child will be unable to receive speech and language services.

A meeting has been scheduled on_____at _____ o'clock, at_____.
At this time_____program will be presented. If you are unable to attend, please contact me at the above circled phone number.

Sincerely,

Speech and Language Pathologist

Figure 5-8. Letter to parents. From West Saginaw County Special Services Area, St. Charles, Michigan.

given. Some of the most popular articulation tests available are listed here.

a. language sample noting articulation errors
b. Fisher-Logeman Test of Articulation Competence (Houghton Mifflin Co.) (Figure 5-9)
c. Goldman-Fristoe Test of Articulation (American

/p, b/	1.	Pete's job was to keep the baby happy.
/t, d/	2.	Today Dick told Patty about it.
/k, g/	3.	The girls were baking the biggest cake for Mr. Tag.
/O, ð/	4.	Their brother wouldn't bathe because he thought a bath would make his toothache worse.
/f, v/	5.	In a half day, he repaired five television sets, two telephones, and a very old stove.
/s, z/	6.	Suzie sewed zippers on two new dresses at Bessie's house.
/ ʃ, ʒ/	7.	She usually rushes to push the garage door closed.
/tʃ, dʒ/	8.	George is at the church watching a magic show.
/r, l, w/	9.	We rode with Lucy around the tall tower in her new yellow car.
/hw, j, h/	10.	Why haven't you looked anywhere behind the house or beyond the hill yet?
/m, n, ŋ/	11.	Nancy found some fine hangers among the many things at the sale.
/i, l, e, ɛ/	12.	Let me keep a little of this wedding cake to eat later.
/æ, a, ɑ, ɚ/	13.	Father asked how much money Tom had saved to buy a bird cage.
/ɔ, o, u, ʊ/	14.	Ruth caught a cold because she wouldn't wear her new warm wool coat.
/aɪ, aʊ, ɔɪ, ju/	15.	I found a huge toy music box outside Roy's house.

Figure 5-9. Sentence Articulation Test of the Fisher-Logeman Test of Articulation Competence (1971). Copyright © 1971 by Houghton Mifflin Company. All rights reserved. Reprinted by permission of Houghton Mifflin Co.

Guidance Service)

d. Developmental Articulation Test (Henja, 1955)

e. Photo-Articulation Test (King Company, 1965)

f. The Templin-Darley Test of Articulation (Templin and Darley, 1960)

g. The "protocol data" sheet checking seven levels of speech by McCabe and Bradley (1973) (see Figure 5-10)

Pre- and postarticulation protocol data sheet from the Cleft Palate and Speech Rehabilitation Program, University of North Carolina Dental School.

Clinician _____   Date_____

Patient _____   Pre _____

Age _____   Post _____

Speaking Modality	Tot. Res.	Tot. Accur.	% Accur.	Text
A				1 2 3 4 5 6 7 8 9 10
B				A B C D E F G H I J K L M N O P Q R S T U V W X Y Z
C				it you for want give is he of to us a the him this they in can car time sit her I one got we let keep down how and that have me use go up cup here there did
D				Name: Address: Age: School:
E				Mamma made some lemon jam. Put baby in the tub. Keep working on the book. Give Gregory the wagon. Show her how to wash the dishes. Suzy saw the sun in the sky. Zippers are easy to close.
F				Title of reading section:
G				Conversation:

Figure 5-10. Protocol Data Sheet. From Robert B. McCabe, *LSSHA School Journal,* Vol. IV, #1, p. 21, 1973.

h. PALST Screening Test (Word Making Publications) 1970

i. McDonald, E.T., A Screening Deep Test of Articulation (1968)

j. Utah Test of Articulation (Communication Research Associates).

THE INITIAL MEETING WITH THE CLIENT

The initial meeting is most effectively carried out in a one-to-one setting. The first meeting should be in an overall relaxed atmosphere and should include a diagnostic study of communication skills of the client. Planning for initial long-range goals can begin at this first meeting.

SUPPLEMENTAL TESTING FOR CLIENTS WITH ARTICULATION DISORDERS

The clinician may wish to probe further into a client's ability in related language areas to predict progress more accurately, and to work more effectively with the total person. Some articulation errors such as /t/ and /ed/ endings and /s/ and /z/ omissions are really language deficits sometimes characteristic of those with mental retardation or hearing loss. Current short supplemental tests include the following:

Peabody Picture Vocabulary Test (Dunn, 1959 and 1965)

Bankson Language Screening Test (Bankson, 1977)

PALST Screening Test (1970)

Riley Articulation and Language Test (1966)

Auditory Discrimination Test (Wepman, 1958)

Boston Discrimination Test (1974)

Check types of articulation errors that might indicate further language problems: *ed, ings, s, z,* endings.

Lengthy supplemental testing is done best by scheduling longer sessions. Other therapists may also assist with this.

SCHEDULING THE CLIENT AND PROGRAM MANAGEMENT

Recent developments in behavior modification techniques have revolutionized management and scheduling of many school programs. The works of the Behavioral Research Institute in Monterey, California, Baker and Ryan (1971), Mowrer (1969, 1978), and many school therapists in Ohio and Michigan have shown good results with the programs emphasizing work with individuals. Individual work was also acclaimed by many of the authors who began speech therapy as a profession (Van Riper, 1937).

Some schools currently insist that there is no room for scheduling individual therapy sessions in a speech clinician's schedule because of the "cost factor." Group therapy still is considered by many to be "cheaper." The facts gathered by Dublinski and Mowrer prove otherwise. Individual scheduling readily appeals to classroom teachers when they see how much less time the pupils spend missing regular classroom subjects.

The following points are scheduling suggestions for a school program based on individual contacts with clients:

1. See every child four days a week for a six to ten week block for a ten to fifteen minute session.
2. Each child knocks on the door of the next child's classroom.
3. Aim for at least five minutes of intensive drill on sound production for the base or transfer stage. Use immediate feedback on every attempt the client makes. Charting and counting may be used to note progress.
4. Challenge the client on his goal and possible criterion before drill begins.
5. Use a minute or two at the beginning to review any homework and a minute or two at the end to assign new work, if appropriate.
6. The clinician uses the remaining few minutes before the next client arrives to record criteria and evaluation of the lesson.

Drill materials from a variety of sources can be used. See the appendix for both programmed materials and workbooks. Client-made lists usually work best for reinforcement.

Programmed materials often need adaptation, and many clinicians prefer to develop their own. Mowrer offers a manual entitled *First Steps in Writing Instructional Programs for Articula-*

tion Improvement. Gerber (1977) gives a good overview of nine such programs and the appendix lists others. Costello (1977) also elaborates on the use of programs.

Use of speech aids in transfer and maintenance stages of therapy should be considered. Former speech pupils and older brothers and/or sisters can do a fine job (Bokelmann and Wallace, 1973).

High school organizations sometimes offer help as do volunteer associations. A paid speech aide might also be considered. Training is needed, however, and aids should be screened for sound discrimination abilities.

The entire staff of a school, clinic, or hospital can be of great assistance if trained. The speech clinician in this approach becomes a "teacher of teachers," extending him/herself in a variety of ways. Informal contacts as well as formal meetings and workshops help. Many classroom teachers are also trained when the school speech clinician does speech improvement sessions in primary grade classrooms.

Parent conferences should be held in addition to the yearly planning meeting. The parents should also observe a demonstration lesson on occasion with their child. Observation of the parents' auditory discrimination skills as well as their abilities to assist should be carefully noted. Many parents need training in auditory skills before they can be of any assistance to their children.

A complete school schedule should be distributed to all as should a summary of the initial screening program at the beginning of the year (see previous section on screening). The printed schedule should include the following:

1. Clients name (correctly spelled) age, grade level, teacher/cottage parent/etc.;
2. Scheduled speech time;
3. Location of client during scheduled speech time;
4. Location of speech room (if this varies during the day);
5. Brief mention of error sound and/or type of problem;
6. Stage of therapy;
7. Times clinician is available for consultation;

8. Names of children to be followed in the classrooms or cottages by the teachers of para-professionals for carryover and maintenance.

Group Therapy

There are many pros and cons to placement of clients in groups. Baird and Clayborne (1974) report that rate of individual therapy success was only slightly higher than group. However, Dublinski (1975) and Mowrer (1973) have collected statistics that found shorter therapy time was required for the children in individual therapy when precision skills and behavior modification techniques were employed than for those children who were placed in group therapy using "traditional" technique. The following items should be considered as scheduling proceeds for groups:

1. Age level and maturity of clients;
2. Attention span of children;
3. Amount of time the child in the group will spend away from a classroom setting, and which class she/he will miss;
4. Time lost while waiting turns in a group;
5. Level and stage of acquisition of the target sound;
6. Possibilities of training group members to assist each other to develop skills;
7. Schedule conflicts and transportation difficulties;
8. Skill of the therapist to deal with various needs of clients within the group;
9. Use of speech aides to assist with the management of larger groups;
10. The need for interaction by clients;
11. Desire and willingness to work in a group.

Actually, nearly all methods and techniques of articulation therapy can be adapted for group use. In a group, the clients often have to wait their turn while the clinician is busy with other children. This often is the main difference between group and individual therapy. It is true, too, that groups can do much for motivation and positive reinforcement, but they can also involve much more time per child to correct a sound as some current research points out. Backus and Beasley (1951) were one of the earliest proponents of a group therapy method based on natural conversational patterns and interaction. Their method is still very usable today. However, if the therapist lacks skills, "group" may resolve into "wait for my turn and be bored" situations.

STEPS IN THERAPY

Choosing a Target Sound

This step involves a complete analysis of a client's sound error patterns. The critical listening ability of the therapist is crucial as is her/his awareness of analysis of patterns of usage of any particular sound.

The following six techniques are important during this more detailed articulation testing process (Winitz, 1975):

1. Listen to the error sounds in conversation and then test further by eliciting with pictures of imitation.
2. Determine any patterns of consistency of errors using many contexts.
3. Search for any contexts where the error sounds are used correctly as a base to generalize production to other contexts.
4. See if the client can imitate the sounds correctly in isolation. If he/she cannot, search other similar phonetic context of sounds.
5. Perform a feature analysis if the client's error sounds are not stimulable in any contexts.
6. Check for consistency in error patterns and see if the errors can be described in terms of any one or two phonetic features.

After these points are considered, it is advised that the clinician narrow the choice of a target sound further with the following steps:

1. The total number and kind of sound errors present should be tallied. The list should be checked to see which sounds are most easily produced in isolation (Milisen, 1954) and which of these misarticulations are consistent. Sounds that

are inconsistently misarticulated and easily produced in isolation will probably be the first choice as rate of success will be high in most cases and will be encouraging to the client.

2. The distinctive features of multiple sound errors should be noted (McDonald, 1964), and the interrelatedness of the features studied carefully (McReynolds and Huston, 1971).

Therapy plans can make use of correctly produced features in many contexts to obtain correct approximations in error sounds. If a number of features are absent, the therapist will want to choose a target sound with a basic missing feature common to the total picture of sound errors.

3. The list of diagnosed errors should be compared with the normal sequence of sounds (Poole, 1934; Templin, 1957; Wellman, 1931; Henja, 1955 and 1960; and Winitz, 1969). A sound produced early in the normal development is usually easily mastered and is a good beginning target sound during therapy.

4. The practical usage and need of the client to use a particular sound is important. For instance, clear production of a word such as a person's name is one of the most important needs of a client. Choosing a difficult sound within a person's name is often highly motivating.

5. The local dialectal patterns of a setting should be noted. The needs and expressed wishes of the clients and/or parents for learning a dialect other than the one spoken in the home should be studied, discussed, and carefully considered. No manner of articulation that is a dialectal property should be condemned or considered inferior in any way. The clinician should carefully analyze the phonetic dialectal differences of his/her locale so he/she is aware that they are not necessarily an articulation disorder. This includes Southern and Applalchian vowel productions, the Boston /R/, the Detroit "twang," as well as the North Dakota consonant voiced/unvoiced substitutions and all the nuances of various black dialects.

Van Riper (1972) also lists some other points to remember when selecting a target sound:
Pick a sound that would—

1. have the most familiar key words.
2. have the simplest muscular coordinations.
3. be mastered earlier by most children in their speech development.
4. be spoken correctly after a bit of trial therapy.
5. have been especially penalized by others in important conversational words.

Establishing a Baseline

Baseline analysis involves precise measurements of a client's competencies at the sound, word, reading, and conversational levels. Use of the conversational sample is advised as the first test. The clinician can record the number of correct/incorrect productions of the specific sound during a three– to five-minute spontaneous speech sample; a tape recorder can be of help, but playback tends to distort some sounds. The errors should be carefully analyzed from the conversation sample. The clinician is advised to continue testing at several other levels as a further probe and check including word lists, reading material (when appropriate), varied nonsense syllables, picture stimuli, words repeated after the therapist, and production of the sound in isolation. Test results should be carefully written down in specific detail at each level.

Another means to record an accurate baseline is use of formal standardized tests. The McDonald Deep Test (McDonald, 1968) is a good example as are pre– and post-tests from a variety of programmed material available commercially and/or developed in many school districts. (See the list of programmed materials in Appendix A: Jackson, 1972; Baker and Ryan, 1971; Smith, 1971; and Diedrich, 1969).

The McCabe and Bradley (1973) protocol test data sheet is also a good general pre– and post-articulation test scheme, which samples all levels of therapy assessment. This scheme is a concise and convenient chart form for use in any therapy setting.

The clinician can always devise her/his own baseline test to focus on the particular stage of articulation skills to be taught. A list of words or sentences repeated after the therapist, picture stimuli, and reading of original connected materials can be used. Shelton has devised (Fig. 5-11) lists of *s, z,* and *r* words useful as a pre– and post-test. Diedrich (1969) has based an entire method of therapy on use of Shelton's list.

It is good to review the sequential development of stages of sound acquisition (Winitz, 1969, 1975). The therapist should be able to ascertain quickly in which of these stages the client is regarding the selected target sound(s). A sample page of objectives in articulation therapy from the Wayne Westland, Bloomfield Hills, and another from the Saginaw Public Schools (Fig. 5-12) shows the sequence outlined in a convenient goal checklist form.

Setting Instructional Objectives

Once the baseline data are collected, the clinician can easily proceed to write out specific instructional objectives. They can be proposed for daily, weekly, semester, and/or terminal lengths of time. This is an important step as it often clarifies goals for all concerned, allows complete program studies for administrators, and allows substitute and student clinicians to easily operate within a program. Public Law 94-142 requires this time. Sample school objectives have been collected by Fairchild and Thomas (1976), and the manuals of many large school speech and language programs are excellent, e.g. Baltimore, Maryland and Cleveland, Ohio (see Fig. 5-13, Detroit).

The method of writing goals varies, but all come to one point: specific statement of the data and how they will be handled. The American Speech and Hearing Association's "PPDME." (Program Planning Development, Management, and Evaluation Workshop Manual) is excellent as are the videotapes presenting the material delivered by Stan Dublinski (1975). Dublinski proposes six components to be stated within a goal: *When?, Who?, What?, To Whom?, Criterion?,* and *Evaluation Methods.* Another method proposed by Mowrer (1976), lists three parts in an objective:

Sound production tasks for /s/ and /z/.

/s/	/z/
1. /us/	1. buzzsaw
2. musty	2. some zest
3. /sae/	3. can zip
4. household	4. does that
5. glass zoo	5. /az/
6. your side	6. big zoo
7. placemat	7. roseland
8. missing	8. /zae/
9. dog sits	9. cheesecake
10. house knife	10. whiz by
11. /s/	11. will Zeke
12. get some	12. /uz/
13. Bob sent	13. Tuesday
14. /sa/	14. beeswax
15. busboy	15. could zebras
16. classday	16. choose him
17. breathe softly	17. wise man
18. clean suit	18. Keep Zoo
19. pass that	19. Take Zeke
20. ice room	20. rose room
21. home soon	21. smooth zebra
22. husky	22. /z/
23. /is/	23. Aztec
24. up Sunday	24. got zero
25. asleep	25. dress zipper
26. his seat	26. Disneyland
27. like soup	27. buzzing
28. all silk	28. Bob zoomed
29. icewater	29. /zi/
30. red socks	30. Her zebra

Sound production tasks for /r/.

1. /ɝ k/ (irk)	31. cooker
2. dear one	32. /gɚg/ (girg)
3. /kru/ (crew)	33. /rɑ/ (rah)
4. /ædɚ/ (adder)	34. /ɛɚ/ (air)
5. girl	35. wrong
6. paper	36. mother
7. rock	37. her
8. /kɝ k/ (kirk)	38. more things
9. /ɪɚ/ (ear)	39. /ri/ (ree)
10. /ɝ/	40. /ugɚ/ (ooger)
11. /gru/ (grew)	41. read
12. beard	42. /dɝd/ (dird)
13. rabbit	43. /ɑɚ/ (are)
14. bird	44. /krɑ/ (krah)
15. /ɑgɚ/ ahger	45. gurgle
16. /tɝ t/ (tirt)	46. brass
17. truck	47. /dri/ (dree)
18. hammer	48. /ɑkɝ/ (ahker)
19. /ræ/	49. crook
20. turn	50. earn
21. gargle	51. /ru/ (rue)
22. /tri/ (tree)	52. /idɚ/ (eeder)
23. /itɝ/ (eater)	53. /grɑ/ (grah)
24. hurt	54. dirt
25. /oɚ/ (or)	55. /træ/
26. /dræ/	56. doorway
27. board	57. ran
28. fur	58. /ukɚ/ (ooker)
29. /ætɚ/ (attar)	59. grey
30. grow	60. shirk

Figure 5-11. Shelton's /s/,/z/, and /r/words. From *Language, Speech and Hearing Services in Schools* by William Diedrich et al., 1969.

do—
conditions—
accuracy—

In either method of writing, the main task of the clinician is to be specific. The more specific the goal, the faster both the client and clinician will move toward it.

Example: Vague goal: Charles will work on the *ch* sound.

Specific goal: Charles will be able to produce the *ch* sound in the initial position in a list of ten words read aloud to the speech clinician with 90 percent accuracy by the end of one week.

SPEECH AND LANGUAGE PATHOLOGY DEPARTMENT
PERFORMANCE OBJECTIVES FOR ARTICULATION DISORDERS

STUDENT_____ AGE_____ BIRTHDATE_____ GRADE_____
ADDRESS_____ PHONE_____ PARENTS_____
THERAPIST_____ TEACHER_____ SCHOOL_____

DIAGNOSTIC EVALUATION:

1. Phonetic Analysis _____   4. Assessment of Discrimination _____
2. Oral Examination _____   5. Other _____
3. Audiological Assessment _____

GOAL: Students will demonstrate improvement or correction in the development of articulation.

UMBRELLA OBJECTIVES: Student will demonstrate improvement in or correct production of phonemes as indicated by 80% correct response measured by formal or informal pathologist evaluation.

UMBRELLA OBJECTIVES	DESIGNATED PHONEME		DESIGNATED PHONEME		DESIGNATED PHONEME		COMMENTS-TECHNIQUES-EVALUATION
SUBJECT WILL BE ABLE TO:	BASELINE	DATE ACCOM.	BASELINE	DATE ACCOM.	BASELINE	DATE ACCOM.	
A. Produce the designated phoneme in isolation.							
B. Produce the designated phoneme in nonsense syllables.							
C. Produce the designated phoneme in the initial position of words.							
D. Produce the designated phoneme in the medial position of words.							
E. Produce the designated phoneme in the final position of words.							
F. Produce the designated phoneme in blends.							
G. Produce the designated phoneme in phrases.							
H. Produce the designated phoneme in sentences.							
I. Produce the designated phoneme in structured conversation.							
J. Produce the designated phoneme in spontaneous conversation.							

Figure 5-12a. Therapy objectives. From *Objectives Checklist in Articulation* by K. Eurich, R. Cunningham, B. Gough, L. Rouhan, and L. Walker. Reprinted by permission of the Bloomfield Hills Schools District, Bloomfield Hills, Michigan.

DEPARTMENT OF PUPIL SERVICES
SPEECH THERAPY DEPARTMENT

NAME_____ AGE_____

SCHOOL _____GRADE_____ TEACHER_____

DIAGNOSIS_____

THERAPEUTIC PLAN:_____

This is a curriculum plan for the remediation and/or amelioration of misarticulated sounds. The following chronological sequence of behavioral objectives is necessary to attain this goal.

DATE
INITIATED

DATE
ACHIEVED
(90% Accuracy)

AUDITORY TRAINING

In speech class the student will be able:

____1. To identify his/her sound when given a sequence of isolated words. ____
____2. To identify his/her speech sound in the initial position of words when given a series of ____ words.
____3. To identify his/her speech sound in the final position of words when given a series of ____ words.
____4. To identify his/her speech sound in the medial position in words when given a series of ____ words.
____5. To discriminate between his/her speech sound and other isolated sounds when given ____ pairs of isolated sounds.
____6. To discriminate his/her speech sound among other speech sounds in words when present- ____ ing a series of words.

VISUAL DISCRIMINATION

In speech class the student will be able to visually recognize and discriminate:

____1. Placement of articulators for his/her speech sound when shown by therapist in isolation. ____
____2. Correct placement of articulators for his/her speech sound when shown by the therapist ____ in word series.

PRODUCTION

In speech class the student will be able:

____1. To tactually identify correct tongue placement for his/her speech sound. ____
____2. To approximate production of his/her speech sound in isolation. ____
____3. To produce correctly his/her speech sound in isolation. ____
____4. To produce correctly his/her speech sound in vowel-consonant combinations. ____
____5. To produce correctly his/her speech sound in words in the initial position. ____
____6. To produce correctly his/her speech sound in words in the final position. ____
____7. To produce correctly his/her speech sound in the medial position. ____
____8. To correctly produce his/her speech sound in blend combinations. ____

STRUCTURED PRACTICE IN CONNECTIVE SPEECH

In speech class the student will be able:

____1. To produce correctly his/her speech sound in prepared phrases. ____
____2. To produce correctly his/her speech sound in prepared sentences. ____
____3. To produce correctly his/her speech sound while reading prepared materials. ____

UNSTRUCTURED PRACTICE IN CONNECTIVE SPEECH

In speech class the student will be able:

____1. To produce correctly his/her speech sound in unstructured sentences. ____
____2. To correctly produce his/her speech sound in conversational speech. ____

Figure 5-12b. Therapy objectives. From "Objectives Checklist in Articulation" by K. Eurich, R. Cunningham, B. Gough, L. Rouhan, and L. Walker. Reprinted by permission of the Bloomfield Hills School District, Bloomfield Hills, Michigan.

School District of the City of Saginaw
Department of Exceptional Services for Children

Review of Objectives

Name_____ Birthdate _____

Program _____ School_____Teacher _____

Date Entered_____

Year End Objectives Articulation: target phonemes_____ _____(Please add objectives re: language, voice, and fluency as appropriate)	October	January	March	May	Comments - Outcomes
_____Consistent auditory discrimination of correctly produced sound(s)					
_____Consistent correct production of sound(s) in isolation and/or short syllables					
_____Consistent correct association of sound(s) with appropriate letters					
_____Consistent correct production of sound(s) in single words					
_____Consistent correct production of sound(s) in short sentences and other structured responses					
_____Consistent correct production of sound(s) during oral reading					
_____Consistent correct production of sound(s) during monitored conversation					
_____Consistent correct production of sound(s) in all speaking situations					

Program Key: 1. accomplished 2. satisfactory progress 3. slow progress 4. little progress

Figure 5-12c. Therapy objectives. From *Objectives Checklist in Articulation* by K. Eurich, R. Cunningham, B. Gough, L. Rouhan, and L. Walker Reprinted by permission of the Bloomfield Hills School District, Bloomfield Hills, Michigan.

DETROIT PUBLIC SCHOOLS

Behavioral Objectives:

1. Given recordings or demonstrations of 10 environmental sounds the learner will identify these sounds through verbal or written response with 90% accuracy.

2. Given a model of the speech mechanism, the learner will correctly name and locate the articulators with 100% accuracy.

3. Given recordings or demonstrations of pitch, intensity, duration or rhythm patterns, or tonal quality, the learner will identify these variations through verbal or written response with 90% accuracy.

4. Given various speech sounds in isolation, syllables, and words, the learner will identify the introduced phoneme with 100% accuracy.

5. Given the incorrect production of the phoneme in isolation, syllables, and words, the learner will identify the correct model with 90% accuracy.

6. Given the correct model, the learner will be able to produce the phoneme in isolation, syllables, and/or words with 90% accuracy.

7. Given the correct model, the learner will correctly produce the phoneme in phrases and sentences with 90% accuracy.

8. Given a reading or story-telling task, the learner will correctly produce the introduced phoneme with 90% accuracy.

9. Given the opportunity for spontaneous speech, e.g. classroom, free play, or home situation, the learner will correctly produce the phoneme with 90% accuracy.

10. Given the opportunity for conversational speech, the learner will correctly produce the phoneme in a follow-up evaluation with 90% accuracy.

Figure 5-13. Behavioral objectives. From *MSHS Journal,* Fall, 1977. Reprinted by permission.

Writing a Terminal Goal

After several weeks of initial therapy, the clinician should once again review the objectives. It is assumed there has been additional supplemental testing and observation of hearing, discrimination skills, language abilities, visual-motor, sequencing skills, and motor abilities during the first sessions and that further study of school achievement and performance in a learning situation has been made. This is the time to write a "Terminal Goal" for the client. A terminal goal states what the client's behavior will be at the end of therapy and estimates the amount of time involved. A well-written terminal goal will list all aspects of speech and language to be remediated and how the client's progress will be evaluated in the final analysis. It can be used effectively in Individual Educational Plan meetings required by the new federal laws for long-range planning. The method of writing suggested is to follow the PPDME (Program Planning Development Management and Evaluation) guidelines and respond to the following six items in this sample:

Date, February 1, 19____

When: By the end of the 4th grade in June of 19____.
Who: Robert Smith
What: Will be able to correctly produce clearly the *ch, sh, l,* and voiced *th* sounds in all positions in words in a 10-minute spontaneous speech sample.
Evaluation: Evaluated by his speech therapist.
To whom: His classroom teacher, peers, and parents will also rate his speech as "intelligible and free from sound errors" in the home and classroom setting. They will be given a rating sheet by the speech pathologist.
Criterion: They will designate his speech as free from errors nearly all the time.

Auditory Training

The clinician should do auditory training during every stage of therapy. Auditory discrimination and memory skills are a vital part of the speech therapy program. The question is not one of should auditory training be done, but rather in what contexts.

Research and study by Mowrer (1973) indicate that the clinician is the first person who needs the "auditory training" in order to deliver accurate feedback to clients. There are sets of commercial tapes to assist clinicians in developing appropriate auditory skills (Mowrer, 1976). The speech clinician can develop his/her own self-training materials by taping lessons and/or co-recording with experienced clinicians.

Some authors advocate auditory training before sound production is taught (Powers, 1971; Eisenson and Ogilvie, 1977; Van Riper, 1972). Other research suggests a speech-defective child's auditory discrimination improves faster when training is concurrent with work requiring mastery of sound production (Mowrer, 1973). These sources reported that auditory training improved faster as a function of teaching the mastery of sound production. Winitz (1977) carefully reviews current studies showing further research needed; he also notes that "phonetic placement" methods are, in fact, 90 percent auditory training because the clinician models the sounds and reinforces client responses. Van Riper and Irwin (1958) also emphasize "self-hearing" of the client in their "scanning and monitoring" approach. They stated that, in a child with defective speech, the tactual and kinesthetic feedback systems are in major control. The clinician's task is to regain the dominance of auditory features in his/her own awareness of speech patterns. "Self-hearing" should be vivid and rewarding, and therefore, should be carefully planned within the therapy lesson. Short, integrated doses can be given. Clients of all ages usually resist lengthy lessons based solely on listening exercises. Lengthy lessons cause disciplinary problems, especially in a group. The clinician can often check the client's auditory awareness by a few simple directives during a lesson and can include other clients in the activity. The most important task is that the client recognize his/her own sound in both his/her own errors and correct productions. Listening to errors in the therapist and in the speech of others is an easier task, and one that can be less challenging. The first and easiest step is recognition of the correctly produced target sound itself in the speech of others. These three items are usually progressively learned, but review of the three simultaneously is necessary.

Use of Audiovisual Material During Sessions

It is important to use all sensory avenues during all stages of therapy. Visual, motokinesthetic, and auditory avenues should all be included as a daily practice routine. Many beginning clinicians tend to stress only one avenue emphasizing only auditory stimulation or relying too heavily on pictures; a good balance of a variety of stimuli is desirable. Especially important is the use of visual aids with self-feedback systems involving motokinesthetic and auditory awareness. A mirror is a must for all stages, as are commercial or hand-drawn pictures. The Floxite Company (Niagara Falls, N.Y.) makes an excellent, mouth-sized magnifying mirror, attaching conveniently to a light; dime stores and beauty counters offer less expensive mirrors.

The client has to learn awareness of the target sound, see the sound, feel the sound, and hear the sound. The clinician's job is to establish the learning atmosphere so the client develops this awareness of production of the correct target sound. Cues from every possible sensory avenue must be used for maximum growth. Books and materials offering diagrams and pictures of the speech articulators include the following:

1. *Phonetics: Theory and Application to Speech Improvement* (Carrell & Tiffany, 1960)
2. *Handbook for Speech Therapy* (Medlin, 1976)
3. *Correction of Defective Sounds* (Nemoy & Davis, 1937)
4. Photo-Phonics Cards (Go-Mo Products)
5. "Form a Sound" cards (Ideal Co.)
6. "Mr. Big Mouth," N.A. Enterprises, P.O. Box 38, Bradford, Mass., 01830.

Training tapes for the clinicians use include the following:

1. "R Discrimination Tapes—Isolation and Context," (Word making Publications)
2. "Evoking Sounds in Young Children" tape (Mowrer, WMP)

STAGES OF ARTICULATION THERAPY

The usual stages of articulation therapy are modeled after the normal sequences of articulation and language development (Winitz, 1969, 1975; Van Riper, 1972). The clinical process can be divided into three steps (Bokelman and Wallace, 1973):

1. Base (teaching sound production and basic words).
2. Transfer (getting the sound itself into all words, phrases and sentences).
3. Maintenance (Carryover).

Gray (1974) outlines similar stages in Baker and Ryan's Monterey Articulation Program, which is said to be "a systematic procedure to teach a student to say a specific sound."

Establishment programs (17 steps, 91 branching steps, sound evocation programs)
Transfer program (15 steps)
Maintenance (5 steps).

Diagnostic testing begins the program, and criterion pre-tests and post-tests are included before and after each stage. Stages sometimes overlap as the client's speech production may be inconsistent, or s/he may be working on more than one sound in advanced stages of articulation therapy.

The Base Stage

Placement in this stage of therapy assumes that the client is not consistent with correct production of a target sound in isolation and/or in words during contact with the clinician. S/he needs to be taught by means including phonetic placement, sound stimulation, tactile, motokinesthetic, and auditory training. The target sound can be taught in isolation and/or by means of a few easy, one-syllable phonetic contexts. Careful testing in a daily pre-test will ensure correct placement at this stage. Accurate discrimination of the target sound and feedback about errors are of paramount importance. Unless the clinician hears the errors and can guide the client in successive approximations towards the target sound, the client will not progress; s/he may, in fact, regress (Mowrer, 1975). Much skill is needed to shape the client's approximations of the sound and judge and reward correct and/or "better" approximations. The following is a list of materials and techniques useful for evoking specific sounds.

1. Mowrer, *Helpbook for Speech Clinicians*, Chapter 2, "Procedures for Evoking Consonant Sounds," 1975.
2. Mowrer, "Evoking Sounds from Young Children" (cassette and text) , 1974.
3. Mowrer, Basic Concepts in Behavior Modification in Speech Therapy, Tape 6, 1975.
4. Nemoy and Davis, *Correction of Defective Consonant Sounds,* 1937.
5. Medlin, *Handbook for Speech Therapy,* 1976.

Establishing the Sound

The first step of therapy should aim at production of twenty successive utterances of the sound during three different sittings. Meetings at this stage may not be formal, if in the school setting. The clinician may wish to make use of lunch time, coordination time, and any chances to see the client briefly in the classroom setting. Clinicians in an institutional, hospital, or clinic setting may wish to train nurses, attendants, and family members to assist at this stage when frequent client contact is not possible. This stage is usually quickly passed if the therapist is competent unless organic problems prevent motor and sensory feedback on the client's part.

As soon as the sound is stabilized, it should be inserted into a syllable, which can then be made into a meaningful word (Jackson, 1972; Winitz, 1975) .

Samples	*Client*	*Clinician*
	er	Good! Now say it again three times.
	er er er	Good! Now hold your tongue still and blow air over it before you say the sound—like this: "her."
	her	Very good. Now say "her hat."
	her hat	Now say "her coat."
	her coat	Good! Now say "her shoe."
	her shoe	Nice! Now whose hat was that?
	her hat	

The sample shows how the new sound is made into a meaningful utterance and lengthened. Words with the /r/ sound are held constant so that at least 75 percent accuracy is achieved. Any task achieving less than three out of four correct responses is too hard and too frustrating for the client. The skillful clinician will adjust to an easier task if 75 percent accuracy is not achieved.

When stabilization of correct production of the sound occurs, the child is ready for the insertion of the sound into words and meaningful contexts. Winitz (1975) also carefully outlines workable procedures for sound production training.

Drill should be expanded to include practice of the target sound in words and phrases. Complexity of the words and addition of sounds in the medial and final positions of words should be developed. The words should be used in meaningful phrases and sentences as soon as possible.

Sample teaching sequence (words repeated after the therapist):

Target sound "l"

/l/ in isolation 1. /l/ in isolation established

/l/ initial 2. /l/ let, leg, like, I like, I like you, leg, leg, big leg, I like, I like you, I like your leg.

/l/ final 3. doll, dolls, dolly, big doll, I like, doll, I like your doll.

/l/ medial 4. yellow, yellow card, like, I like, I like your yellow card. doll, dolly, I like your dolly. Does the dolly have yellow hair?

/l/ sounds 5. little, little, doll, little boy, little doll, like, I like your doll, little, I like your little doll.

spontaneous 6. Now tell me about the little doll with yellow hair.

Notice there is constant review of previous materials. Also note the consistent use of the same key words in vocabulary. Of course, these six stages may take many sessions to develop, but sometimes, in minor cases with older clients, they can be completed in one session.

When enough drill is accomplished to build up use of the target sound up to 80 percent accuracy during reading words or

80 percent in highly structured speech class activities, the Transfer Stage has been reached.

Sources for programmed materials for the Base Stage include the following:

1. Costello, Programmed Instruction, 1977.
2. Psaltis and Spallato, *Programmed Articulation Therapy,* 1972.
3. Jackson, /R/ and /Sh/ Program (WMP), 1972.

Essentially "Traditional Therapy," Backus and Beasly," "Paired Stimuli," and Van Riper all involve the *Base Stage.* It is the skill of the clinician that makes any method succeed.

Transfer Stage

This is begun after the client has at least 80 percent success of use of a target sound in a structured speech setting and can read the sound successfully with 90 percent accuracy. Transfer programs aim to establish stable use of a target sound with 100 percent accuracy during conversation in the presence of the speech clinician or other trained para-professionals. Since the actual teaching of sound production has been successfully completed at this stage, the use of speech aides and other para-professionals can be well utilized to extend the program and to develop and strengthen carryover and maintenance skills. They must be well-trained and be under the direct supervision of the master clinician (Committee on Supportive Personnel, ASHA, 1969; Perry, 1973).

Again, correct discrimination of the target speech sound and immediate feedback to the client are of direct importance. The client now uses the target sound in more difficult words, phrases, sentences, and connected structured speech. Continued feedback is given by the clinician and/or aides, but criterion is higher. When errors drop below 4 percent, more teaching at the base stage may be needed; the clinician should then be directly called upon for teaching assistance. Many games and activities can be used at this stage. Therapy can be individual or group as the client's needs and the setting indicate. Clients can be trained to assist one another and to count errors and give feedback. Winitz (1975) outlines a number of transfer techniques. Programmed materials are also available for a number of sounds (see Appendix A).

Maintenance Stage

The client is now to the point that s/he uses the target sound with 100 percent accuracy in the speech class setting in all situations, especially spontaneous conversation. However, it is still noted by family, peers, teachers, and staff that the client makes a few noticeable sound errors outside speech class. The clinician can train many of the child's contacts to note errors and can ask them for feedback on progress. A simple rating sheet is often effective (see Fig. 5-14). Wing and Hemgartner (1973) offer a systematic program for maintaining correct use of a sound. It involves parent, guardian, or trained aides, and has five levels. It may be done in the home setting under supervision of the clinician. The five levels are summarized:

1. 100% mastery of use of the target sound in a ten minute reading during three successive sessions. The parent counts and charts while the child reads. This counting and charting is followed for all 5 levels.

2. 100% mastery of the target sound during a 5 minute reading followed by 5 minutes of questions given by the recorder. Three successive 100% accurate sessions are expected.

3. The client and parent/aide talk together for 10 minutes while client's errors are recorded and charted. After three successive 100% successes, step 4 is undertaken.

4. The parent/aide selects 10 minutes during a given hour to record and chart clients errors. After three successive 100% accurate sessions, step five is begun.

5. The parent/aide selects 10 minutes, in 1–10 minute segments during a day to record. The client does not know at what time the charting and counting are being done. After three successive counts, the client is offered congratulations and given a "conditional" dismissal certificate.

It is assumed that the client will be checked periodically for possible regression for a year or two before final dismissal is made. Selection of clients for this type of structured "maintenance" program should be carefully made as cooperation of parents, guardian, or aides must be obtained.

Other authors have indicated methods and materials suitable for the Maintenance Stage (Mowrer, 1971; Miller, 1971; Wing and Heimgartner, 1973; Winitz, 1975). The clinician who blames the client instead of setting up a systematic plan can be suspect of not understanding the total learning process.

CLASSROOM TEACHER'S EVALUATION OF
SPEECH PROGRESS

Child's Name   Teacher's Name

Grade   Please return to the speech
                                       therapist by _____

Diagnosis

Improvement of Speech   Speaking
    When Reading
    1. no improvement   1. no improvement
    2. slight improvement   2. slight improvement
    3. considerable improvement   3. considerable improvement
    4. inconsistent   4. inconsistent
    5. other   5. other

Yes   No   Errors on the _____ sound are very noticeable
             during classwork.

Yes   No   Errors on the _____ sound are slightly notice-
             able during regular class work.

Yes   No   No errors on the _____ sound are noticeable in
             classroom work.

Remarks:

                              Signed_____

                              Date _____

Figure 5-14. Teacher's rating sheet. From Speech Therapy, Putnam County, Ottawa, Ohio. Originated by Sister Marie Kopin.

THE "OLDER" CLIENT IN A SCHOOL SETTING

Persons who are over ten years old who have articulation disorders usually require careful program management by the clinician. Pupils in school settings who are in the fifth, sixth, seventh, and eighth grade may highly resent leaving class settings and be wary of peer ridicule. Establishing rapport with teachers and other school personnel is very important in educating students to the worth and benefits of speech in an upper elementary and junior high school setting. The clinician can do much by working with language arts teachers on a consultative basis. These teachers are most often eager to cooperate because speech-disordered students usually have other associated language problems. Teachers' advice, recommendations, and classroom materials can be of valuable assistance. The therapist should strongly consider incorporation of classroom assignments as materials for clinical sessions. The senior high school student may prefer to take speech remediation for high school credit, or as a regular part of English class given individually. Sometimes it is also a prudent measure to schedule after or before school hours as well as during study halls. Again, education of the total school staff and especially the language arts teachers is necessary for a successful program.

Materials for older clients should be geared to their level. Goda's book, *Articulation and Consonant Drill Book* (1970), is good for advanced readers; Schoolfield's *Better Speech and Better Reading* (1937) has useable lists for lower grade levels. The Detroit Board of Education also publishes materials for the advanced reader.

CLIENT MOTIVATION

It is important to keep the client motivated. Accurate feedback and correct selection of stages of therapy are necessary. An "aware" client can make decisions to improve her/his speech, while one who is constantly "being told what to do" and being told "you didn't work hard enough" by a therapist employing a parental approach may rebel. The clinician can review the specific instructional objectives with the client so there is common agreement on what therapy is all about. Charting and counting help in recording progress in a concrete fashion so the client can see day to day progress (Mowrer, 1971; McCall, 1973; Diedrich, 1969). Periodic reports to parents are helpful (see Fig. 5-15).

SPEECH THERAPY PROGRESS REPORT TO PARENTS

Name_____ School_____ Date_____

Difficulty_____

Sound (s) and/or problem being stressed at the present time: _____

Progress:

    1. Produces the sound   Sometimes_____ Yes_____ No_____

    2. Uses the sound in words   Sometimes_____ Yes_____ No_____

    3. Uses the sound in sentences   Sometimes_____ Yes_____ No_____

    4. Uses the sound in reading material Sometimes_____ Yes_____ No_____

    5. Uses the sound in conversation   Sometimes_____ Yes_____ No_____

    6. Almost ready for dismissal   Sometimes_____ Yes_____ No_____

    7. Cooperates with speech therapist   Sometimes_____ Yes_____ No_____

    8. Works well with the other children Sometimes_____ Yes_____ No_____

    9. Shows a desire to improve speech
        through own efforts   Sometimes_____ Yes_____ No_____

   10. Needs to practice more outside the
        speech class   Sometimes_____ Yes_____ No_____

Additional Comments:

    I would appreciate hearing any suggestions, questions or comments you may have concerning your child's speech. Please feel free to contact me at your convenience. The space above is provided for any written comments you may have. Would you please sign and return this at your earliest convenience.

                              Sincerely,

                              _____

                              Speech and Hearing Therapist

                              _____

                              Parents Signature

Figure 5-15. Progress report.

The condition of the therapy room is also an important factor. Even the darkest corner can come alive with the help of an imaginative therapist. One clinician in the Cleveland Public Schools, who was placed under a dark stairwell, made a "speech cave" and used ordinary school supply paper to decorate it accordingly; the children could not wait to come to her.

MATERIALS AND THE SPEECH NOTEBOOK

Materials are available from a number of publishers and sources. In the 1970s, several companies began to cater more to needs in special education including speech therapy. Appendix A includes a list of suppliers. "Clinician-made Materials" are good, but are time-consuming for the professional. Clients can also be encouraged to prepare their own materials during therapy sessions.

Use of a speech notebook can be beneficial to communicate with family and to encourage carryover activities. A good speech notebook should include the following:

1. Name of client, age and/or grade level, address, teacher's name, time of speech session.
2. Simple pictures and instructions on production of the target sound (Nemoy and Davis, 1937, Goda, 1970).
3. A message to parents (staff, spouses, etc.) on what the book is and what is expected of them.
4. An attractive cover and contents to appeal to the appropriate age level of the client.
5. Every page should have clear instructions on its use.

RECORDS

It is mandatory that the speech clinician keep careful records of the progress of each client. Recording a simple tally after each session, even if only an estimate of the lesson's content and success and/or failures, will enable the clinician to draw up a comprehensive evaluation of his/her program. Several sample charts are to be found in Figure 5-16.

Client time in therapy can be recorded and then compared for self-study and program improvements. Comprehensive reports of

NAME ______________________ CLINICIAN ______________________

DATE ______________________

STRUCTURE ______________________
SC ______________________
EXPANSION ______________________

1								
2								
3								
4								
5								
6								
7								
8								
9								
10								

Percent Correct ________

STRUCTURE ______________________
SC ______________________
EXPANSION ______________________

1								
2								
3								
4								
5								
6								
7								
8								
9								
10								

Percent Correct ________

Structure ______________________
SC ______________________
Expansion ______________________

1								
2								
3								
4								
5								
6								
7								
8								
9								
10								

Percent Correct ________

Structure ______________________
SC ______________________
Expansion ______________________

1								
2								
3								
4								
5								
6								
7								
8								
9								
10								

Percent Correct ________

Structure ______________________
SC ______________________
Expansion ______________________

1								
2								
3								
4								
5								
6								
7								
8								
9								
10								

Percent Correct ________

Structure ______________________
SC ______________________
Expansion ______________________

1								
2								
3								
4								
5								
6								
7								
8								
9								
10								

Percent Correct ________

Figure 5-16a. Data collection sheets, by Kathleen Stremel-Campbell. Reprinted by permission.

NAME————————

DATE————————

SESSION Na————————

CLINICIAN————————

DATE	TRIALS/ITEMS	TASK																							
		1	2	3	4	5	6	7	8	9	10	11	12	13	14	15	16	17	18	19	20	21	22	23	24	25

SUMS/MEANS

COMMENTS:

Figure 5-16b. Data collection sheets. From Putnam County. Originated by Sister Marie Kopin.

services rendered also impress administrators and provide "ammunition" for obtaining more clinicians, better cooperation, and better facilities and supplies. Careful records are also extremely helpful in the required IEP meetings mandated by Public Law 94-142.

EVALUATING PROGRESS . . . THE CLIENTS AND THE CLINICIANS

The final step of the management of clients with articulation difficulties is an evaluation of the total program by the clinician. How many clients have reached termination? How long did it take them? Which methods and techniques proved most successful in a particular clinical setting? Can any result of the evaluation be shared with other staff and other speech pathologists? What new techniques could be tried next year? Were parents, spouses, and other professionals, agencies, and peers satisfied?

In such a self-study of a program, helpful directions for improvement can come to light as well as enough facts and figures to impress supervisors, taxpayers, boards, and government agencies of the effectiveness of programs and needs for further development.

NO SPEECH PATHOLOGIST STANDS ALONE

Again, this is a comforting thought and one of the underlying principles of this chapter. The clinician works with parents, other clinicians, peers, and many professionals of all kinds. None of these individuals is likely to be trained in communication disorders; thus there are great potential and opportunities to educate these fellow workers. A good speech program should include many people, who can teach articulation skills in conjunction with their everyday interactions with articulation-defective children. A few minutes well spent by the clinician at the school or hospital cafeteria, before school, during coffee breaks, in phone calls, and in formal speaking engagements and conferences can round out the total program and assist in developing a speech-oriented staff in a school, clinic, or hospital. The enthusiastic positive attitude of a speech pathologist can permiate an entire program. Pamphlets and books can be made available in teacher's lounges and libraries. Family members also usually want to help; an older brother or sister can be trained to assist in the schools. Parents often appreciate the opportunity to attend a "Teach a Child to Talk" workshop or at least read a handbook (Collins, 1977). Provision for a simple speech notebook or workbook with homework exercises provides not only appealing work to show parents but can also serve as a source of communication to the home and a reminder to practice and review material.

No speech clinician ever stands alone; this may seem questionable at times, but in reality, individuals with speech and language problems are everyone's concern and responsibility.

References

American Speech and Hearing Association: *Program Planning Development, Management, and Evaluation Workshop.* West Lafayette, Ind., Purdue, 1974.

Backus, O. and Beasley, J.: *Speech Therapy with Children.* Boston, Houghton Mifflin Co., 1951.

Baird, S.M. and Clayborne, D.: The effectiveness and efficiency of group and individual therapy for articulation disorders in a public school setting. *J TN Speech Hearing Assoc, 18 (2):*13-15, 1974.

Baker, R.D. and Ryan, B.P. *Programmed Conditioning for Articulation.* Monterey, California, Monterey Learning System, 1971.

Baltimore County Board of Education: *Speech, Hearing and Language Therapy,* A resource manual. Towson, Md., 1971.

Bankson, N.: *Bankson Language Screening Test.* Baltimore, Md., University Park Press, 1977.

Blomquist, B.L.: Diodochokinetic movements of nine, ten and eleven year old children. *J Speech Hearing Dis, 15:*159-164, 1950.

Bokelmann, D. and Wallace, E.: *Training speech aides to administer five transfer programs.* Short Course at ASHA, Detroit, 1973.

Boston Discrimination Test. Cedar Falls, Iowa, Go-Mo Products, 1974.

Brandell, M.E., Robertson, J.H., and Piotrowski, P.: *The /R/ Control Kit.* ASHA Convention Presentation, Washington, D.C., 1975.

Brown, J.C.: Techniques for correcting /r/ misarticulation. *Lang Speech Hearing Serv Schools,* VI:86-91, 1975.

Brown, R.: *A First Language, The Early Stages.* Cambridge, Mass., Harvard University Press, 1973.

Carrell, J. and Tiffany, W.R.: *Phonetics: Theory and Application to Speech Improvement.* New York, McGraw-Hill Book Co., 1960.

Chicago Board of Education, Division of Speech Correction: *Speech Correction Techniques and Materials* (revised). Chicago, 1952.

Collins, N.: *Teach Your Child to Talk, A Parent Handbook.* CEBCO/ Standard Publishing Co., 104 Fifth Ave., New York, N.Y. 10011, 1977. Also producers of the Workshop Kit, *Teach a Child to Talk.*

Committee on Supportive Personnel, ASHA: Guidelines on the role, training and supervision of the communication aide. *Language Speech*

Hearing Serv Schools. 1:48-53, 1969.

Costello, J.: Articulation instruction based on distinctive features theory. *Language Speech Hearing Serv Schools,* VI:61-71, 1975.

Costello, J. and Onstine, J.M.: The modification of multiple articulation errors based on distinctive feature therapy. *J Speech Hearing Dis, 41:* 199-215, 1976.

Costello, J.M.: Programmed instruction. *J Spech and Hearing Dis, 42:* 199-215, 1976.

Costello, J.M.: Programmed Instruction. *J Speech and Hearing Dis, 42:* 3-28, 1977.

Delbridge and Larrigan: *Stimulus Shift Articulation Kit.* Ideas, information, dissemination, exchange and service, Tempe, Ariz., 85281, 1974.

Diedrich, W.M.: Procedures for counting and charting a target phoneme. *Language Speech Hearing Serv Schools, 1,* 18-32, 1969.

Dublinske, S. Analyzing the clinical process. Speech at ASHA Convention, Washington, D.C. 1975.

Dunn, L.: Peabody Picture Vocabulary Test. American Guidance Service, 1959 and 1965.

Eisenson, J. and Ogilvie, M.: Defects of articulation; Treatment of articulatory difficulties. In: *Speech Correction in the Schools,* 4th ed. New York, Macmillan, 1977, 263-305.

Fairchild, L. and Thomas, C.: A public schools subcommittee report, Samples of performance objective form, etc. *J of the Michigan Speech and Hrn Assoc, 12:*147-162, 1976.

Fisher-Logeman Test of Articulation Competence, Geneva, Ill., Houghton Mifflin, 1971.

Flowers, A.: *The Big Book of Sounds.* Cedar Falls, Iowa, Go-Mo Products, 1966.

Gerber, A.: Programming for Articulation Modification. *J Speech Hearing Dis, 42:*29-43, 1977.

Goda, S.: *Articulation Therapy and Consonant Drill Book.* New York, Grune and Stratton, 1970.

Goldman-Fristoe Test of Articulation. Circle Pines, Minn., American Guidance Service Pub., 1969.

Gray, B.: A Field Study on Programmed Articulation Therapy. *Language Speech and Hearing Serv in Schools. V:*119-131, 1974.

Harryman, E. and Kresheck, J.: A structured program for modifying /r/ misarticulations, *Language Speech Hearing Serv Schools, 1:*52-57, 1969.

Hatten, J. and Laroque, D.: Changing directions in public speech therapy. *Ohio J of Speech and Hearing, 7:*15-22, 1972.

Hejna, R.F.: *Developmental Articulation Test.* Madison, Wis., College Printing and Typing, 1955.

Hejna, R.F.: *Speech Disorders and Nondirective Therapy.* New York, Ronald Press, 1960.

Irwin, J.V.: *Modification of Articulatory Behavior by the Paired Stimuli Technique,* Short Course at ASHA, Chicago, 1971.

Irwin, J.: The Triota: A computerized Screening battery. *Acta Symbolica, 3:*26-38, 1972.

Irwin, J.V. and Weston, A.J.: *The Paired Stimuli Technique.* Memphis, Tenn., National Education Services, 1971.

Irwin, R.B. and Becklund, O.: Norms for minimum repetitive rates for certain sounds established with the sylrater. *J Speech Hearing Dis, 18:* 149-160, 1953.

Jackson, M.: *R Correction Program and SH Correction Program.* Tempe, Ariz., Word Making Productions, 1972.

Kuly, J.L., Madison, C.L., and Prather, E.: *Articulation and Speech Sound Perception of Primary-Age Children for the Phoneme /s/.* Paper presented at ASHA, 1973. Detroit, Michigan.

Keller, F.: *Learning Reinforcement Theory.* New York, Random House, 1954.

Knox, J.: *Knox Articulation Correction Program.* Tempe, Ariz., Ideas Corporation, 1976.

Lubbert, L., Johnson, Brenner, and Alderson: *Behavior Modification Articulation Program for Speech Aides.* Tempe, Ariz., Ideas Corporation, 1974.

Maxwell, K.: *A comparison of certain motor performances of normal and speech defective children, ages seven, eight, and nine years.* University of Michigan. Ph.D. dissertation, 1953.

McCabe, R. and Bradley, D.: Pre- and Postarticulation Therapy Assessment. *Language Speech Hearing Serv Schools, IV,* 13-22, 1973.

McCall, E.: Making progress in speech correction more visible. *Language Speech Hearing Serv Schools, IV:*45-46, 1973.

McDonald, E.T.: *Articulation Testing and Treatment: A sensory-motor approach.* Pittsburgh. Stanwix House, 1964.

McDonald, E.T.: *A Screening Deep Test of Articulation.* Pittsburgh, Stanwix House, 1968.

McReynolds, L. and Engmann, D.: *Distinctive Feature Analysis of Misarticulation.* Baltimore, University Park Press, 1975.

McReynolds, L.V. and Huston, K.: A distinctive feature analysis of children's misarticulations. *J Speech Hearing Dis, 36:*155-166, 1971.

McReynolds, L., Engmann, D., and Demmitt, K.: Markedness theory and articulation errors. *J Speech and Hearing Dis, 36:*155-66, 1971.

McReynolds, L.V. and Bennet, S.: Distinctive feature generalization in articulation training. *J Speech Hearing Dis, 37:*462-470, 1972.

Medlin, V.L.: *Handbook for Speech Therapy.* Salt Lake City, Word Making Productions, 1976.

Messich, L.: *Through My Day with the S, R, L, SH Sound.* Palo Alto, Calif., Pacific Books Pub., 1971.

Milisen, R.A.: A rationale for articulation disorders. *ASHA Monogr, 4:* 5-18, 1954.

Miller, D.: *Carryover Articulation Manual.* Springfield, Thomas, 1971.

Mowrer, D.E.: *Basic Concepts of Behavior Modification in Speech Therapy.* (Cassette) Salt Lake City, Word Making Productions, 1975.

———: *Behavior Modification Techniques with School Children Who Have an Articulation Disorder.* Speech at Columbus, Ohio, May, 1973.

———: *Developing Precision in Recording Speech Behaviors.* Salt Lake City, Word Making Productions, 1976.

———: *Discrimination Training Program for "er."* (Cassette and booklet) Salt Lake City, Word Making Productions, 1975.

———: *Evoking Sounds from Young Children.* Salt Lake City, Word Making Productions, 1974.

———: *First Steps in Writing Instructional Programs for Articulation Improvement.* Tempe, Ariz., Information, Dissemination, Exchange and Service, 1975.

———: *Helpbook for Speech Clinicians,* Tempe, Ariz., Arizona State U. Bookstore, 1975.

———: *Lectures in Methods of Speech and Therapy.* Tempe, Ariz., Arizona State U. Bookstore, 1970.

———: *Modification of Speech Behavior; Ideas and Strategies for Students.* Tempe, Ariz., Arizona State U. Speech Dept., 1969.

———: *Transfer of Training in Articulation Therapy. J Speech Hearing Dis, 36:*427-446, 1971.

Mowrer, D.E., Baker, R.L., and Schutz, R.E.: *Modification of the Frontal Lisp Programmed Articulation Control Kit.* Tempe, Ariz., Educ. Psychol. Res. Assoc., 1968.

Mowrer, D.E., Baker, R.L., and Schutz, R.E.: S-Pack, S. Programmed Articulation Control Kit. Tempe, Ariz., Ideas Corporation, 1970.

Mysak, E.D.: *Speech Pathology and Feedback Theory.* Springfield, Ill., Thomas, 1971.

Nemoy, E.M.: *Speech Correction Through Story Telling Units.* Magnolia, Mass., Expression Co., 1958.

Nemoy, E. and Davis, S.: *Correction of Defective Consonant Sounds.* Magnolia, Mass., Expression Co., 1958.

PALST Screening Test (articulation and language): Salt Lake City, Word Making Publications, 1970.

Perry, J.: Iowa: *Profile of a Speech Aide.* Paper at ASHA, Detroit, MI, 1973.

Photo Articulation Test. Chicago, The King Company, 1965.

Pollack, E. and Rees, S.: Disorders of articulation; some clinical applications of distinctive feature theory. *J Speech Hearing Dis, 37:*451-461, 1972.

Poole, I.: Genetic Development in articulation of consonant sounds in speech. *Elem Eng, II:*159-161, 1934.

Powers, M.H.: Clinical and educational procedures in funational disorders of articulation. In Travis, L.E. (Ed.): *Handbook of Speech Pathology and Audiology.* New York, Appleton-Century-Crofts, 1971.

Precision, Teaching, Special Child Publication. 4535 Union Bay Place N.E., Seattle, Washington 98105, 1976.

Programmed Articulation Skill Carryover Stories. Tucson, Ariz., Communication Skill Builders, 1976.

Psaltis, C.D. and Spalatto, S.L.: *Programmed Articulation Therapy; Time to Modify.* Springfield, Ill., Thomas, 1973.

|R| Articulation Modification Program. C.C. Publications, P.O. Box 372 Gladstone, Oregon, 1976.

Riley, B.: Riley Articulation and Language Test. Western Psychological Services, Box 775, Beverly Hills, California, 1966.

Schenfield, D.D.: *Games Kids Like.* The Learning Business Inc., Westlake Village, California 91361, 1974.

Schoolfield, L.D.: *Better Speech and Better Reading.* Magnolia, Mass., Expression Co., 1937.

Scott, L.B. and Thompson, J.J.: *Talking Time.* New York, McGraw-Hill, 1951.

Scripture, M.K. and Jackson, E.: *A Manual of Exercises for the Correction of Speech Disorders.* Philadelphia, Davis Co., 1927.

Schriberg, L.D.: A response evocation program for *J Speech Hearing Dis, 40:*92-101, 1975.

Sloane, H. and MacAulay, B.: *Operant Procedures in Remedial Speech and Language Training.* Boston, Houghton Mifflin Co., 1968.

Smith, R.M.: *The R—Sound Workbook.* Johnstown, Pa., Mafex Associates, Inc., 1971.

Somers, R.K. and Kane, A.R.: Nature and remediation of functional articulation disorders. In Dickson, S. (Ed.): *Communication Disorders; Remedial Principals and Practices.* Glenview, Ill., Scott, Foresman and Co., 1975.

SWRL Program for Articulation. American Book Company, Div. of Educational Research and Development, Lampson Ave., Los Alamos, California 90720, 1973.

Templin, M.: *Certain Language Skills in Children.* Minneapolis, U of Minn Pr, 1957.

Templin—Darley Tests of Articulation. Bureau of Educational Research and Service, Division of Extension and University Services, University of Iowa, Iowa City, 1960.

Tjomsland, L.: *Feel it and Say it.* New Richmond, Wis., Whitehaven Pub. Co., 1968.

Toohey, D.: *Precision Speech Explored.* Workshop presented, September, 1975, Ohio.

Van Riper, C.: *Speech Correction; Principles Methods,* 1st, 5th, and 6th ed. Englewood Cliffs, Prentice-Hall, Inc., 1937, 1972, 1978.

Van Riper, C., and Irwin, J.V.: *Voice and Articulation.* Englewood Cliffs, Prentice-Hall, Inc., 1958.

Waters: *Articulation Base Programs for K-G; F-V; and SH.* Dept. of Comm. Dis., Northern Ill. University, DeKalb, Ill. 60115, 1975.

Wellman, B., Case, I., Mangert, I., and Bradbury, D.: *Speech Sounds of Young Children.* University Iowa Studies in Child Welfare, 5, No. 2, 1931.

Wepman, J.: Auditory Discrimination Test. Chicago, Language Research Associates, 1958.

Weston, A.J., and Irwin, J.V.: Use of paired stimuli in modification of articulation. *Percept Motor Skills, 32:*947, 1973.

Williams, G.M.: *A Systematic Behavior Approach of Prevision Therapy.* Fairfield County Schools, Lancaster, Ohio, 1973.

Wing, D. and Heimgartner, L.: Articulation carryover procedure implemented by parents. *Language Speech Hearing Serv Schools, 4:*182-195, 1973.

Winitz, H.: *Articulatory Acquisition and Behavior.* New York, Appleton-Century-Crofts, 1969.

Winitz, H.: *From Syllable to Conversation.* Baltimore, University Park Press, 1975.

Winitz, H.: Articulation disorders; From prescription to description *J Speech Hearing Dis, 42:*143-147, 1977.

Writing Individualized Programs. Workbook for Speech Pathologists. Gladstone, Oregon, C.C. Publications, Inc., 1976.

Young, E. H. and Stinchfield-Hawk, S.: *Moto-Kinesthetic Speech Training.* Stanford, Stanford Pr, 1955.

APPENDIX A

PUBLISHERS AND RESOURCE MATERIALS

PUBLISHERS of Material Useful for Articulation Therapy
and Speech Sound Stimulation Exercises
for Clients of All Ages

American Guidance Service, Inc., Publishers Building, Circle
Pines, Minn. 55014

Appleton-Century-Crofts, New Centura, 440 Park Avenue South,
New York, New York 10016

Arizona State University Bookstore, Arizona St. U., Tempe,
Arizona

Barnell Loft, Ltd., Dexter, and Westbrook, LTD, 958 Church St.,
Baldwin, N.Y. 11510

Bobbs-Merrill Company, 4300 West 62 Street, Indianapolis,
Indiana 46268

Bowman Publishers, 622 Rodier Drive, Glendale, California
91201

Charles C Thomas, Publisher, 301–327 East Lawrence Ave.,
Springfield, Illinois 62717

Charles E. Merrill Publishing Co., 1300 Alum Creek Drive,
Columbus, Ohio 43216

C. C. Publications, P. O. Box 372 Gladstone, Oregon

Cleo Living Aids, 3957 Mayfield Road, Cleveland, Ohio 44121

Communication Skills Builders Inc., 817 East Boradway, Tucson,
Arizona 85733

Constructive Playthings, 1040 East 85th Street, Kansas City, Missouri 64131

Developmental Learning Materials, 7440 Natchez Avenue, Niles,
Ill. 60648

173

Educational Activities, Box 392, Freeport, New York 11520

Educational Teaching Aids, A Daigger & Co., Inc., 159 W. Kinzie St., Chicago 60610

Educator Press, Box 444, Monterey, California 93940

Educators Publishing Service, 75 Moulton St., Cambridge, Mass. 02138

Expression Company, Magnolia, Mass.

Fearon Publishers/Lear Siegler, 6 Davis Drive, Belmont, Calif. 94002

Floxite Company, Inc., P.O. Box 1094, Niagara Falls, N.Y. 14303

Follett Educational Corp., 1010 West Washington Blvd., Chicago, Ill. 60607

Garrard Publishing Company, 2 Overhill Rd. Scarsdale, N.Y. 10583

Ginn and Company, A Xerox Education Co., 191 Spring St., Lexington, Mass. 02173

Go-Mo Products, 1906 Main Street, Cedar Falls, Iowa 50613

Holcomb's Educational Mart, 3000 Quigley Rd. Cleveland, Ohio 44113

Holt, Rinehart and Winston, 383 Madison Ave., New York, N.Y. 10017

Ideal School Supply Company, 11000 S. Lavergne Av., Oak Lawn, Ill. 60453

Ideas, P. O. Box 741, Tempe, Arizona 85281

Instructo Corporation, Cedar Hollow & Matthews Road, Paoli, Penn. 19301

Interstate Printers and Publishers, 19–27 N. Jackson St., Danville, Ill. 61832

Learning Business, 30961 Agoura Road, Westlake Village, Cal. 91361

Learning Concepts, 2501 N. Lamar, Austin, Texas 78705

Macmillian Company, 866 Third Avenue, New York, N.Y. 10022

Mafex Associates, Inc., 90 Cherry Street, Box 519, Johnstown, Pa. 15907

Milton Bradley Company, Springfield, Massachusetts 01101

New York Times Teaching Resources, 100 Boylston Street, Boston, Mass. 02116

Northwestern Univ. Press., 1735 Benson Ave., Evanston, Illinois 60201

Oddo Publishing, Box 68, Fayetteville, Georgia 30214

Opportunities for Learning, 5024 Lankershim Blvd., Dept. A7, N. Hollywood, Calif. 91601

Pacific Books Pub. P. O. 558, Palo Alto, Calif. 94302

Prentice-Hall, Educational Book Division, Englewood Cliffs, New Jersey 07632

Phonovisual Products Incorporated, P. O. Box 5625, Washington, D.C. 20016

(The) Psychological Corporation, 75/Third Avenue, New York, N.Y. 10017

Scholastic Magazines & Book Services, 50 W. 44 St., New York, N.Y. 10036

Scott Foresman and Co., 1900 E. Lake Avenue, Glenview, Ill. 60025

Stanwix House, Inc., 3020 Chartiers Ave., Pittsburg, Penn. 15204

SWRL Education Research and Development, American Book Co., 4665 Lampon Ave., Los Alancitos, Calif. 90720

Teaching Resources Corporation, 100 Boylson Street, Boston, Mass. 02116

Trend Enterprises, Box 3073, St. Paul, Minn. 55165

University of Illinois Press, Urbana, Illinois 61801

University Park Press, Chamber of Commerce Bldg., Baltimore, Md. 21202

Webster Publishing Co., St. Louis, Mo. 63155

Western Pub. Co., Educational Division, 850 Third Avenue, NY, NY. 10022

Western Psychological Services, 12031 Wilshire Blvd., Los Angeles, Calif. 90025

Whitehaven Pub. Co., Inc., Box 2, New Richmond, Wis. 54017

Word Making Products, 60 West 400 South St., Salt Lake City, Utah 84101

Resource Materials for Articulation Therapy

1. *Through My Day with the S, R, L, and SH Sounds.* Pacific Books Co., 1972.

2. "Procedures for Counting and Charting a Target Phoneme," *Diedrich, Lang, Speech and Hearing in Schools,* 1969.
3. *Carryover Articulation Manual* (developed by UCLA Speech Clinic) Charles C Thomas Pub. or Opportunities for Learning Co., 1976.
4. *Speech Correction Through Story Telling Units,* Expression Co. 1958.
5. *Correction of Defective Consonant Sounds,* Nemoy and Davis, Expression Co., 1937.
6. *Handbook for Speech Therapy,* Medlin, Word Making Products, 1976.
7. *Programmed Articulation Skills Carryover Stories,* Communication Skill Builders, 1976.
8. *Programmed Articulation Therapy: Time to Modify,* Psaltis and Spalloti, Charles C Thomas, Pub., 1973.
9. *Games Kids Like* and *More Games Kids Like,* The Learning Business Inc., 1974.
10. *Better Speech and Better Reading,* Schoolfield, Expression Co., 1937.
11. *Talking Time* and *Speech Ways,* Scott, Webster Pub. Co., 1951.
12. *Speech Correction Techniques and Materials* (revised), Chicago Board of Education, 1952.
13. *Speech, Hearing, and Language Therapy,* A Resource Manual. Board of Education, Baltimore County, Md.
14. *Feel it and Say it,* Jomsland, Whitehaven, 1968 (Motokinesthetic Method), 1975.
15. *Articulation Base Programs for K-G; F-V; and SH,* Waters, Northern Ill. U. Press, 1975.
16. "Articulation Carry over Procedure Implemented by Parents," *LSHSS,* 1973.
17. *Behavior Modification Articulation Program for Speech Aides,* Lubbert et. al., Ideas Corporation (cassette tape and text).
18. *Knox Articulation Correction Program.* This program is for clinicians or speech aides. Ideas Corporation.
19. *The Big Book of Sounds,* Go-Mo Products.

20. *SWRL Speech Articulation Kit,* SWRL Education Research and Development, American Book Co. This is a structured program for /s/, /l/, /th/, and /r/ sounds using a speech aide and supplemental home work by parents.
21. *A Systematic Behavioral Approach of Precision Therapy,* Fairfield County Schools, Lancaster, Ohio, 1976.
22. *Helpbook for Speech Clinicians,* Mowrer, 1975, Arizona St. University Bookstore.
23. Baker, R.D. and Ryan B.P.: "The Montery Articulation Program." Montery Learning Systems, 99 Via Robles, Monterey, California 93940.
24. Strong, B.N.: "Articulation Program for Technicians." Coordinator of Speech Therapy, Public Schools, Thief River Falls, Minnesota 56701.
25. Diedrich, W.: "Procedures for Counting and Charting a Target Phoneme." *Lang Sp Hear Ser Sch,* 1, 18-42; 1969.
26. *Listen-Hear* (1964) and *Junior-Listen-Hear Books,* (1968) Slepian and Seidler, Follett Pub.
27. Goldman-Lynch, *Sounds and Symbols,* Story Books 1 and 2 (for Speech Improvement) American Guidance Service, 1971.
28. *My Speech Workbook* Series, Parker, 1961, The Interstate Publishers.
29. *Talking Magic,* Marquardt 1965, The Interstate Publishers (for Speech Improvement).
30. *Flethers* drill game, Educator Press.
31. *"SH" Correction Program,* Jackson, Word Making Productions, 1976.
32. "Blazhz" game, Whitehaven Pub.
33. *Best Word Book Ever,* Scarry, Western Pub. Co., 1974.

Specific Materials and Techniques for Stimulation of the /R/ Sound

1. *The /R/ Control Kit.* ASHA Convention Presentation, Brandell, Robertson & Piotrowski, D.C., 1975.
2. "Techniques for Correcting /r/ Misarticulations," Brown, *LSHSS,* 1975.

3. "A Structured Program for Modifying /r/ Misarticulations," Harryman & Kresheck, *Lang Sp Hear Ser Sch,* Vol. I, 1969.
4. "Procedures for Counting and Charting a Target Phoneme," Diedrich, *Lang Sp Heart Ser Sch,* 1969.
5. */R/ Correction Program,* Jackson, 1972, Word Making Productions.
6. *Discrimination Training programs for /r/* (cassette & booklet) , Mowrer, Word Making Publications.
7. "A Response Evocation Program for /r/ "Schriberg, *J Sp Hear Dis,* 40, 1975.
8. *The /R/ Sound Workbook,* Smith, Mafex Associates, 1971.
9. *The Correction of Defective Consonant Sounds,* Nemoy and Davis, Expression Company, 1954, 140-320.

Specific Materials and Techniques for Stimulation and Teaching of the /S/ Sound

1. *Modification of the Frontal Lisp Programmed Articulation Control Kit,* Educ. Psychol. Res. Assoc. (1968) and Word Making Publications.
2. *Stimulus Shift Articulation Kit for /s/ and /z/ distortions for Clinicians and/or trained aides,* Ideas Corporation, 1976.
3. *S-Pack,* S Programmed Articulation Control Kit, Mowrer, Ideas Corporation.
4. "Utilization of the Straw Technique for Correction of the Lateral Lisp," Usdan, *Lang Sp Hear Serv Sch,* IXCI, 5.7, 1978.
5. *The Correction of Defective Consonant Sounds,* Nemoy and Davis, Expression Company, 1954, 149-346.

Chapter 6

STUTTERING

Leslie Gruber

To the Clinician

T HIS CHAPTER IS BEING WRITTEN primarily to the clinician, who is
involved in the day to day challenge of improving the speech
of the person who stutters and in the evaluation and treatment of
the condition of stuttering. Many clinicians have expressed the
concern that they feel less adequate in working with stuttering
than with most other speech and language disorders. The material that follows is designed to present the stutterer in a more
humanistic fashion and thus modify some of the negative precon-
ceptions and misconceptions you may have about becoming involved with those persons who stutter, who so desperately need
help.

In your readings, discussions, and lectures concerning the onset
and development of stuttering, you were probably introduced to
statements such as stuttering is a bad habit and could be broken
if the stutterer just had enough will power, or stuttering is a
manifestation of an arrest at the oral or anal stage of sexual development or, stuttering results from the misperceptions and
evaluations of a child's environment. Or, stuttering occurs because of a defect in an individual's perceptual feedback system
or that it is an expressive problem brought about by cortical
malfunctioning resulting in perseverative behavior. Or it is a
conditioned response resulting from intermittent reinforcement.
And on and on and on went the philosophizing, theorizing, and
hypothesizing.

No doubt these sometimes conflicting, erudite, and awesome

theories left you feeling confused, lost, and inadequate in your abilities to cope with the situation when you suddenly realize you would have to confront and interact with a fellow human being who might possess some of these characteristics. Were you not pleasantly surprised and relieved when you introduced yourself to your client, said "Good morning, how are you?" to him, and this supposedly oral-anal, misevaluated, intermittently reinforced individual with the defective feedback mechanism answered, I-I-I-I-I-I'm fine a-a-a-a-and how are y-y-y-y-y-you."

The Stutterer's Feelings

Although many of the theories about stuttering are conflicting and do create confusion and uncertainty, you must ultimately deal with a human being who has a communication problem. You may be dealing with a child who is not even concerned about how he talks but whose parents and teachers may be worried. Or, you may be working with a teenager or an adult who is deeply concerned about his speaking difficulties and is looking for help and guidance. He is looking for someone who he feels understands his problem and will help him find a satisfactory solution for it. He will want to talk about how his palms sweat or how butterflies flit to and fro in his stomach or how his heart pounds when he hears a telephone ring or even when he just thinks about having to make a phone call. Or, his concern may be the reason why he cannot push his words out or why his lips tremor when he tries to make a *p* sound.

Doing the Wrong Thing

Always remember that when you first meet your client you know more about stuttering than he does. You may feel that your intervention will jeopardize your client because you might do THE WRONG THING. That phrase has been used to cover up a multitude of insecurities and inadequacies by the professional in training and even those of us who have been in the field for decades. I would not be too concerned about that if I were you since we still do not know what THE RIGHT THING is. Certainly there are times when you are going to do THE WRONG

THING and will probably do it many times. You are dealing with human interactions, and even that rare personage in our culture called a wise man sometimes does the wrong thing. Besides, stutterers are not hothouse plants. Peacher and Harris (1947) showed that, in war, combat stutterers as a group were remarkably tough. They have known mistreatment all their lives. They have been rejected because of how they talk. Parents, wives, and sweethearts are sometimes embarrassed by their stutterers. Sometimes the stutterer is mocked and laughed at. Eyes turn away and heads are bowed as he begins to struggle to speak his thoughts. Yet, the majority of stutterers continue to try to interact with their fellow human beings, to grow up, marry, have children, and complain about their taxes. In short, despite maltreatment and mistreatment, the stutterer attempts to stumble and muddle his way through life, solving his problems the best he can just as his normal speaking brothers and sisters do. In you he is not going to encounter many of the rejections he meets in daily life. He is going to encounter a human being who is learning to keep eye contact as he meets another human being in trouble. You are not going to mock, laugh, or reject him. In you he will see someone who cares and who is trying to understand, sometimes agonizingly so. The stutterer will respond almost instinctively. He is hungry for someone who will accept him with all his blemishes, and this you surely can provide for him. Also, do not be afraid to reveal your own feet of clay. It will only make you seem more human.

Helping the Stutterer

Do not do the stutterer the injustice of treating him like a person who is going to fall apart, explode, or collapse if you do the wrong thing. Explore his stuttering with him. Put his struggle behavior into your mouth and show him that the feeling of being stuck does not have to lead to feelings of fear and helplessness. Show him that a tight, tense, blocked mouth can be unblocked and that smooth transitions can be made from one sound to the next. Show him that he does not have to thrash around in the throes of his helplessness but can stutter in several ways, one of them in a more relaxed, less tense fashion without his habitual avoidance and release mechanisms. In short, share the stutterer's experience with him. Give him support as he tries out new ways of responding in different types of situations. Help him to tackle the situation of which he has always been afraid. In most cases, when a stutterer realizes the effort you are putting forth, he will appreciate it. Once he realizes that you care and are trying to help him, you will find that you can do many things wrong without jeopardizing his chances. He will feel that you are a person who can be trusted. So, take your anxieties, concerns, and insecurities in hand and begin to explore some of the things that can be done to evaluate and treat the stutterer.

ASSESSMENT OF THE YOUNG STUTTERER

Speech Evaluation

Many times in your professional career you will be called upon to evaluate the speech of a young child in order to determine whether or not he is a stutterer. More than one teacher or parent is going to approach you about a particular child and will say "I think Johnny is a stutterer and should have therapy." What will your answer be? Upon what basis are you going to make your decision? Or, you may encounter the reverse situation, in which you listen to the speech of a child and think he is stuttering but no one in the environment is acknowledging the condition. What criteria would you use to determine whether a problem exists? Following is a discussion of disfluencies in general and some specific guidelines for evaluating disfluencies in terms of stuttering behavior.

Types of Disfluencies

A great deal has been written concerning the speech development of young children. It is agreed that most children, as they are in the process of acquiring their language skills, exhibit disfluencies in their speech. Words, phrases, and sentences do not pop out of a child's mouth ready-made when he learns how to talk. He stumbles, hesitates, and repeats as he progresses in his language development. When the young child becomes an adult, he will continue to exhibit disfluencies although not as frequently. He will continue "er, uhm" repeat and stumble throughout his life, for there is not a human being who can speak perfectly at all times.

Johnson (1959) delineated several different disfluencies including repetitions of sounds, syllables, words, phrases, prolongations, interjections, revisions, and broken words, which he found in normal speaking children as well as in children who were considered stutterers. Perhaps it is this fact that has led some authorities to deny the existence of the primary, phase one, incipient, or whatever term may be chosen to designate the child who is beginning to stutter, and to conclude that all disfluencies exhibited by children were normal.

Stuttering Disfluencies

There is considerable controversy concerning those behaviors which should be labeled as stuttering. Although all children do exhibit many different types of disfluencies, are there specific types that serve to designate stuttering? Van Riper (1971) believes that there are and that they consist of the repetitions of sounds and syllables. He believes that, if a child exhibits these repetitions in sufficient quantities, the child will likely become labeled a stutterer. If the word is fractured too often and a child's speech is sprinkled with this type of behavior, so that when he wants a glass of water he says "m-m-m-mommy may I-I-I-I-I ha-ha-have a glass of w-w-w-w-water," ten environmental ears become alerted, and he is in danger of being called a stutterer. In contrast, authorities such as Johnson (1959) and Shames and Sherrick (1963) feel that since normal speaking children also exhibit stutterings these behaviors should come under the rubric of normal disfluencies and that a child should not be considered a stutterer until he begins to react to his disfluencies with struggle, tension, and avoidances.

To resolve this controversy, it appears that we need to answer the question of how much stuttering is considered normal. How many stutterings can a child reveal before he is in danger of being labeled a stutterer? For an excellent evaluation and discussion of the stuttering–normal nonfluency controversy, the reader is referred to the writings of Wingate (1962) and Bloodstein (1975), who seem to support the classic study of Davis (1939) .

DAVIS'S STUDY. It is this writer's opinion that no study has investigated the status of repetitions of young children as thoroughly as Davis; her article will be discussed here. Davis investigated the instances of repetitions in the speech of sixty-two children ranging in age from twenty-four through sixty-two months or roughly between the ages of two and five. Only one of the children in this group was considered a stutterer. Her findings indicate that preschool children repeat on the average forty-five times per thousand words—a figure that has since been quoted many times to support the contention that all children repeat as they learn their speaking skills. Her breakdown of repetitions, however, according to length of linguistic utterance, has seldom, if ever, been mentioned. Her study indicated that forty-two of the forty-five instances of repetitions consisted of word and phrase iterations, while only three of the repetitions consisted of syllabic iterations.* In addition, approximately one-quarter of the children did not repeat any syllables, thus refuting the contention that all children have this type of repetition, while another one-quarter of the children had one or two repetitions per thousand words. Thus, for approximately half of her subjects, syllable repetitions were a rare occurrence. However, every child, except one, had word repetitions while all children had phrase repetitions. The repetitions of words and phrases decreased with age while syllable iterations remained constant across age levels. The one child in her study who was considered a stutterer did not differ from his contemporaries in terms of word and phrase repetitions but did differ significantly in terms of syllable repetitions. He evidenced sixty-six repetitions per thousand words, which was 12.4 standard deviations above the mean.

It would appear that syllable repetitions are somehow "different" from word and phrase repetitions and that it is this type of behavior that should be your major diagnostic tool in attempting

---

*Syllable repetitions refer only to part-word or nonmorphemic repetitions, such as bu-bu-butter. They do not refer to one-syllable, whole-word repetitions such as and-and-and.

to reach a decision on whether a child should be considered a stutterer.

Not only the instances of repetitions but the number of repetitions per word appear to determine when the environment begins to use the terms *stuttering* and *stutterer* as shown in Sander's (1963) study. He concluded that instances of double-unit repetitions such as Sa-Sa-Saturday evoked more stutterer judgments than twice the same number of single-unit repetitions such as Sa-Saturday, indicating the sensitivity the environment has towards this type of behavior.

CONCLUSION. As a rule of thumb, if a child has more than twenty instances per thousand words of syllable repetitions (taking into consideration the variation that occurs among normal speaking children), and if the repetitions contain several of the triple-unit or greater variety, then you should not treat this child as a normal speaking child but rather as a primary stutterer.

FURTHER CONSIDERATIONS. During the evaluation of the young stutterer, you must be alert to the behaviors that a child may be showing other than easy repetitions of sound and syllable. The speech of a stutterer changes over time, and as he becomes older his symptoms change form in the direction of greater severity. Talking becomes increasingly difficult.

Symptom Changes

The additional symptoms the stutterer acquires include prolongations, hard contacts, excessive tension, tremors, extraneous movements of face and body, and avoidance behaviors including substitutions, postponements, and circumlocutions. In addition, the stutterer's feelings towards the communication process also change. During the early stages of stuttering, he is not concerned about the bobbles in his speech. With the passage of time this unconcern changes to feelings of frustration, surprise, unpleasantness, and finally to embarrassment, shame, guilt, fear, and anxiety. Further, the situational factor must be evaluated. Has the stutterer become cued in to specific types of situations? Does the stutterer shy away from speaking on the telephone, talking before his peers in a group situation, or ordering a meal in a restaurant? Thus the factors of overt speech, covert attitudinal behaviors, and situation anxieties must be evaluated if an intelligent plan of therapy is to evolve.

Classification

You, the therapist, must determine where on the continuum ranging from beginning to chronic severe stuttering your particular child belongs. In classifying your stutterer, the use of the Van Riper (1963) traditional classification of primary, transitional, and secondary stuttering may be combined with his current 4 track system (1971). His traditional system is valuable as a guide to determining whether therapy should be environmental, indirect, or direct as described by Luper and Mulder (1964). A discussion of each of these types of therapy will be presented in a subsequent section.

The 4 Tracks

The 4 track classification will increase your awareness of the differences that may exist within stutterers. Not all stutterers stutter for the same reason, nor do they evidence the same symptoms during the onset and development of this disorder. Thus, therapy for all stutterers cannot be the same.

Track I describes the stutterer you are most likely to find in your case load and who has the best prognosis during the course of treatment (Van Riper, 1971). His stuttering usually starts between two and one-half and four years of age after he has had a period of fluency. His major stuttering symptom consists of the easy, bubbly repetitions of sounds and syllables. These repetitions are regular, blend in with the prosodic features of his utterances, and are cyclic in nature. He may go for days, weeks, or months without any noticeable stuttering when suddenly the symptoms appear, then disappear again only to reappear. He may have three or four of these on again–off again periods. When the child is fluent, he is very fluent. He seems to enjoy talking, and many times his parents complain that he talks all the time. He is not concerned with his disfluent speech and evidences no frustration or fear. He is generally of normal intelligence with good aritculation and language. As the stutterer grows older, his symptoms increase in severity. Repetitions become irregular, prolongations enter, hard contacts begin followed by tremors and, finally, avoidance devices. His feelings change from pleasure to surprise to frustration and finally to fear. His stuttering becomes predictably associated with specific types of situations. Speech ultimately becomes full of "Jonah" words and situations, and communication becomes a terrifying experience.

Track II differs from track I in that the child never was fluent, was delayed in language, and began to stutter as soon as he began to talk. Articulation is poor, and stuttering symptoms such as gasps, fast spurts, and repetitions appear. As this stutterer grows older, the frequency of his symptoms changes but their form remains essentially the same. He evidences few avoidances and does not develop the intense fears of the track I stutterer. Van Riper (1971) claims that this stutterer has occasional fears of situations but not of words or sounds.

The track III stutterer forms only a small minority of the stuttering population. His stuttering begins suddenly and dramatically, and his parents have no difficulty in pinpointing when they first noticed their child stuttering. From the beginning he has much tension, laryngeal blockings, and tremors in contrast to the easy repetitions of the track I stutterer. His symptoms are consistent. He is highly aware of his stuttering, presents the most morbid picture, the strongest fears, and the most marked avoidances of the stuttering children.

The children in track IV also form a small minority of stutterers. They seem to gain some neurotic reward from their stuttering and use it as a means of controlling their environment. They generally begin stuttering later than the children of the other three groups. Van Riper (1971) describes their stuttering as being deliberate and controlled. It is unique from the beginning with bizarre facial and bodily mannerisms such as biting, tongue and lip protrusions, or wide-open jaws accompanied by retching noises.

It becomes obvious that a careful case history, particularly concerning the onset of a child's stuttering, must be taken if you are to understand his problem and intelligently form a plan of therapy for him.

SITUATIONAL EVALUATIONS

The evaluation of a child's speech should be done in as many different situations as possible, including his speech performance both at home and in school. This information may be obtained from tape-recorded samples, clinical interview with the parents, and from observation and discussion with the classroom teacher.

Speech Performance at Home

A great deal of information concerning the child's speech performance in different situations can be obtained from the parents. During an interview, it is preferable that both the mother and father be present. As you explore the child's speaking performance at home, demonstrate the type of behavior you are trying to identify. Not only describe the disfluency you are evaluating, but *show* it. If you are demonstrating the easy type of repetitive behavior, the repetitions will seem to blend in with the prosodic features of the sentence. Their pitch, intensity, and inflectional patterns will flow along with the rest of the sentence. If, however, you are demonstrating the tense type of behavior, the repetitions are irregular, and forcing is evident. You actually seem to be blocked in the forward flow of speech.

Variability of Stuttering

Explain to the parents that their child's stuttering may fluctuate in different situations. He may stutter less in communicating with one person than another with whom he feels less at ease. He may stutter more during a classroom situation than in spontaneous yelling on the playground. Ask the parents to describe a typical day in the life of their child, identify the different situations he encounters and whether they have noticed that he has more difficulty in talking in one or more of them. If the parents are vague in this matter, have them keep a log of the times that their child seems to be having noticeable difficulty and to record what the immediate environment was doing and saying at that time. Was the child fighting for competition to talk at the dinner table? Was he being asked to explain his behavior and did father seem angry while asking for this explanation? Did he show more stuttering when he went to visit his grandparents?

Parental Correction of Speech

Explore the ways in which the parents have tried to help their child talk. Do they do a great deal of correcting? Are they constantly stopping his forward flow of speech to have him say a word over again? Through public education, many parents have learned not to draw their child's attention to the speaking process. They have been told to say nothing to him when stuttering is manifested and to accept this manner of speaking. If they follow these instructions, they are told, the speaking apparatus will mature, and the child will eventually obtain normal speech. This is sound advice, but you must also explore whether parental acceptance of a child's stuttering is nonverbal as well as verbal.

Facial and Body Cues

Many times parents will convey their anxiety and concern by means of nonverbal behavior, such as facial and body language. For example, the analysis of one parent's body language revealed that, everytime her child began to exhibit strings of repetitive verbal utterances, she would hold her breath. The child began to notice this intermittent breath holding and ultimately associated this behavior with the stutterings occurring in his mouth. Thus, repetitions and breath holding became related. Another parent exhibited concern by frowning, while a third parent raised her eyebrows.

The impact of nonverbal behaviors may be counteracted by first becoming aware of them and then replacing them with more positive expressions. Breathing can be made to flow normally, smiles can replace frowns, and eyebrows can be lowered.

Speech Performance at School

Much information can be obtained concerning the child's speech through communicating with his classroom teacher. Often it is the teacher who first makes the diagnosis that the child is stuttering and refers him to the therapist. You should always evaluate the child's speech in the particular stituation in which the teacher has noticed his having difficulty. Was it during oral reading, spontaneous speaking before his peers, reporting to the principal, or simply talking to the teacher on an individual basis? By observing the child in his actual disfluent situations, you and the teacher can discuss and come to an agreement concerning the child's speech behavior. Differences of opinion can thus be prevented.

Therapist-Teacher Conflict

The following situation can arise if exchange of information between you and the teacher is accomplished by notes or by classroom, hall, or coffee room conversation instead of actual observation. A child may stutter severely in a large group situation such as the classroom but may be fluent in a one-to-one or small group situation such as therapy. If a teacher sends the child to you, claiming he stutters, and you tell the teacher that her diagnosis is incorrect—that he does not have a stuttering problem—your credibility diminishes rapidly, and rapport and cooperation with the classroom teacher, which are so essential to the stutterer's well-being and progress, are lost.

Classroom Teacher Input

The teacher can be a fruitful source of information, providing insight into the child who stutters. She observes the child in many different types of situations and can specify those in which he is relatively fluent and those in which he exhibits speech difficulty. This input is important to exploit the child's fluent periods by praising him and building up his self-worth and to arrange his "trouble situations" in a hierarchy according to degree of difficulty. Many suggestions for teacher participation in the therapy process may be found in the writings of Johnson et al. (1967), Egland (1970), and Eisenson and Ogilvie (1977).

Academic Performance

The classroom teacher is helpful in providing you with knowledge concerning the stuttering child's academic performance. Areas of academic strengths and weakness can be determined to effectively incorporate language skills into the therapy plan. Specific techniques to accomplish this will be discussed in the therapy section.

Communication Attitudes

You can learn of the child's attitude towards talking in various situations from his classroom teacher. Does he seem tense and anxious when she calls the roll and he is expected to answer "Here" or "Present?" During show and tell time, does he seem eager to participate? When reading aloud, does he appear frustrated, ashamed, or embarrassed when he cannot read smoothly?

In summary, it becomes evident that teacher-therapist interaction contributes a great deal of insight into a child's speaking and emotional make up, which is essential in developing a therapy plan tailored to his specific needs.

THERAPY FOR THE YOUNG STUTTERER

Therapy for the young stutterer may be environmental, indirect, or direct, depending on his symptoms. If he exhibits easy repetitions of sounds and syllables and appears unconcerned about them, environmental therapy is generally considered appropriate. If the child is in the early transitional stage of stuttering where he is beginning to show some awareness of his difficulties, and his speech pattern is changing form such as bursts of irregular repetitions appearing or the "siren" effect occurring in his prolongations, then the indirect form of therapy would be the chosen procedure. At this stage, the child may refer to himself as a stutterer, but the word does not seem to have much meaning to him. Someone may have uttered this word in his presence, and he just seems to be repeating it. He has not yet incorporated the word *stutterer* into his ego structure and seems unconcerned about the fact his environment may consider him as such. When the child approaches the end of the transitional stage, exhibiting excessive tension in the use of his oral musculature and forcing out his words; when he starts to use nonverbal secondary devices such as eye closures and loss of eye contact or verbal avoidances such as postponements and substitutions; when he reacts to his difficulties with obvious distress and frustration, then the first or second level of direct therapy as described by Luper and Mulder (1964) is the logical choice. The third level of direct therapy is generally reserved for the older child and adult chronic secondary stutterer and will be discussed in a subsequent section.

Environmental Therapy

Environmental therapy implies no direct contact between therapist and child. Your role consists of being a source of information and a counselor to parents and teachers in attempting to identify and reduce any pressures that advertently or inadvertently are being placed upon the child. You attempt to insure that talking remains a pleasant experience for him without any emphasis being placed on his disfluent behavior.

Environmental Pressures

In his excellent chapter concerning the treatment of the beginning stutterer, Van Riper (1973) discusses some of the relevant pressures that need to be considered, identified, and if possible, reduced and eradicated. These pressures include punishing and calling attention to a child's stuttering. The parents are advised not to correct the speech of their child and are given a list of "don'ts" with which most therapists are familiar.

Another one of the major disruptors to communication is listener loss. If this factor is evident, you must train the parent to become a good listener. This writer remembers only too well the case of four-year-old primary stutterer who exhibited a great deal of nonfluent behavior in the presence of his father. The father was a high-powered executive who used his home primarily as a place to hang his hat, be fed, and sleep between meetings. He never had any time for his son, and the child was always trying to gain the attention of his father when he was either entering or leaving the house in a hurried flurry of activity. The pressure placed upon the child was so great that it resulted in speech breakdown. Fortunately, the father cared for his child, and, when it was pointedly explained to him that it was his behavior that was creating the stuttering, a compromise situation was reached.

Every day for a half-hour period after supper, the father belonged to the child. They talked, played on the floor, and engaged in co-operative activities. The father found this helped him to wind down from the day's pressures and began to extend the play periods with his child whenever time permitted.

You must be warned, however, that not all counseling sessions end this successfully, but at least you must try to produce changes in the home environment of a stuttering child whenever the situation appears warranted. Sometimes the parent, usually the father, does not want to attend these counseling sessions. He is not interested in taking advice from some fresh-faced female just out of college or from any female for that matter. Also, in many situations, specific pressures cannot be identified. Either the parents will not cooperate in analyzing their own behavior, or the child may have such an unstable speaking mechanism that even pressures that might be considered slight or innocuous set off his stuttering.

Other pressures that may cause fluency breakdowns are constant interruptions and competition during communication. In some homes, verbal bandits are in evidence everywhere. The moment a child hesitates or stumbles in his speech, he has lost the conversation ball. In this situation, it is sometimes efficacious to hold a conference with the entire family, preferably without the young child being present. At this meeting, the deleterious effect of the family's behavior can be explained and a plan formulated to provide the young stutterer with the security that, once he begins to talk, he will be able to finish what he intended to say.

Active Parental Participation

It is useless to tell parents not to worry about their child's stuttering. Parents have always been concerned or worried about their children and will continue to be so. Instead of constantly advising what not to do, it is more helpful to show them what they *can* do. Parents are constantly asking, "What can we do to help our child?" One suggestion is to ask the parents to accept their child's current way of talking as being normal for him; the stumblings he is revealing will decrease as he gets older. If he finds talking joyful and rewarding, he has an excellent chance of gaining normal speech. Generally, the young stutterer enjoys verbal interaction with his environment. In fact, many parents state that his speaking patterns do not bother him, that he talks all the time, and that they sometimes find his verbal diarrhea annoying. This admission provides you with the opportunity of having the parents realize the importance of fostering a positive attitude towards talking and accepting the child's speech the way he does. It is often more advantageous if the parents emulate the attitudes of their child. A technique to accomplish this is to ask a series of questions. In this way, the parents gain insights by themselves rather than having you provide them with all the answers. Self-insights are most effective. If their child is truly a happy child, the following series of questions may bring the parents to this realization. (1) Does Johnny enjoy talking to people? (2) Does he enjoy talking to both children and adults? (3) Has he any friends? (4) Does he enjoy playing with his friends? (5) How does he like school? If the parents answer yes to the above questions, you can summarize by stating that Johnny appears to be basically happy and emotionally healthy child who happens to have some bobbles in his speech.

Slow Down

You can also provide the parents with some interactive techniques to be carried out in the home. One of these would involve slowing down the child's emotional and speech behavior. Several authorities have noticed that a child often exhibits more disfluencies in his speech when he is excited (Luper and Mulder, 1964; Van Riper, 1971; and Bloodstein, 1975). This excitement places greater demands on the speaking mechanism and may overload its electrical circuitry, causing misfirings and resulting in the oscillatory behavior we call stuttering. By having the child slow down, an opportunity is provided for the stabilizing of neuromuscular activity and normal speech results. Some authorities state that a child should not be told to slow down since this will only cause him to become aware of his speech. This writer does not subscribe to this point of view. Shearer and Williams (1965) and Sheehan and Martyn (1966), in exploring the spontaneous recovery of stutterers, reported that in the majority of cases the former stutterers claimed that their parents telling them to slow down was the major factor in their spontaneous recovery. It is certainly not advocated that every time a child stutters he be told to speak slower but that the slowing down directive should be aimed at his overall emotional behavior and not only towards his mouth. If he has seen a bird swoop down from the sky and has run excitedly into the house to tell his mother about it and begins to stutter, she should slow down his overall behavior. In doing so his speech will automatically become slower.

A good activity that parents can share with their child to create a relaxed, unhurried atmosphere is "slow motion speech or lazy speech." This type of speech can be combined with nonverbal behavior. For example, mother and child may walk slowly around the room naming and talking about objects, performing both the walking and talking in slow motion or lazy fashion. Or, they may flop down on the sofa like rag dolls and lazily communicate with each other from this position. Or a chair in the house may be designated as the lazy talking chair. Anybody sitting in that chair must drag out sounds.

Pseudostuttering

Another technique to prevent any negative attitudes that may arise is to train the parents to occasionally stutter voluntarily to their child. The type of stuttering to be performed is the relaxed repetition of syllables with no more than two or three repetitions per word, something like th-th-this. Mother can either say, "Oops, I stumbled on that word," or simply smile and continue talking, or evidence no reaction at all. Thus, by example, she sets a positive attitude towards this type of disfluency. This pseudostuttering need not be shown more than three or four times in the course of a day. These are but a few of the suggestions that may be given to enable the parents to play a more active role in helping their child learn to talk more easily.

Indirect Therapy

For the beginning transitional stutterer, the indirect approach is recommended. Indirect therapy implies direct contact between

child and therapist.   The child is seen on a regular basis for the
sole purpose of providing him with pleasurable speaking experiences.   No attention is focused on his speech.   He may engage
in a one-to-one relationship with you, or he may be placed in a
small group situation where he talks about his favorite topics,
such as his pet dog, TV programs, or his beloved grandparents.
Or, as Luper and Mulder (1964) suggest, play groups may be
organized and creative dramatics instituted based upon the child's
interests.

Direct Therapy

The first and second levels of direct therapy are usually reserved for the transitional stutterer as he is nearing the end of this
stage.   At the first level, the emphasis is on speech improvement
with no mention made of the stuttering.   The child is not aware
that you are working at decreasing his disfluencies.   With this
type of therapy, the procedures are more structured than with the
indirect form.   Activities such as choral reading and rhythmic
speaking are suggested.   During choral reading, both you and the
child read or talk in unison, and then you gradually fade out of
the picture until the child is reading solo.   If he begins to evidence stuttering, you reenter the situation until he is talking
fluently and then repeat the process of fading out.   Rhythmic
speaking will be described in therapy for the older stutterer.

The second level of direct therapy is aimed at the child who is
highly aware of his stuttering but has not developed the complex
symptomatology of the more advanced stutterer.   His struggle is
acknowledged, and the symptoms are catalogued but not discussed
in great detail.   The emphasis is placed on learning to talk more
easily.   Gross secondary escape mechanisms such as eye closing or
pronounced lip postures are brought to the child's attention, and
he is encouraged to talk without them but not forced to analyze
or "face" them.   This would only leave him feeling miserable.
With his avoidance techniques or tricks such as "er" or "uhm"
used as a postponement device before a difficult word, a more
frontal attack is recommended.   Following are some suggestions
to achieve the goals of identification and elimination of these
symptoms.

Catch Me

Van Riper (1973) advocates the "Catch Me" game to have the stutterer learn what he does that prevents him from talking easily. First the behaviors to be eradicated are identified. Then you and the child take turns at deliberately inserting them into your speech and catching each other. Children usually enjoy this procedure especially if rewards are introduced and if they win more than you do. This serves to counteract any unpleasantness they may have attached to their avoidances.

Finally, the "Catch Me" technique is useful to have the child discriminate between hard and easy stuttering. First he identifies your stuttering as hard or easy and then you categorize his voluntary blocks. After this discrimination has been accomplished, the child classifies his own real stutterings.

The Stuttering Apple

A device for structuring therapy and identifying maladaptive behaviors is suggested by Cooper (1965). A graphic representation termed the stuttering apple is used to present the problem in concrete terms. A small circle is drawn to depict the core of the apple, and words such as *blocks* or *getting stuck* are written in this circle to indicate the basic problem. Then the symptoms that you and the child discover forming a part of his stuttering repertoire are written in small circles, which you attach to and surround the core. Cooper suggests that terms such as *I blink my eyes* or *I jerk my hand* or *I don't answer in class* should be inserted into the circles instead of words such as *expectancy, nonfluency, avoidance,* and *anxiety.* Thus, the stutterer's problem is presented in a vocabulary he understands. Once the behaviors to be eliminated are identified, he is told that he is now going to take bites out of the apple, implying that he is to try to eliminate the symptom depicted in the selected circle. When he has eliminated all the circles around the core, it will disintegrate and fall apart.

Rewarding Stuttering

Language learning can be combined with stuttering therapy and serve to help the child acquire a healthier attitude towards his disfluencies. First, consult with his classroom teacher and select an appropriate reading passage. Tell him that you are thinking of a word in that passage, that he is to try to guess it, and provide him with its first sound in a repetitive fashion. For example, if you are thinking of the word *run,* repeat the *r* sound several times (r-r-r-r-r) while the child scans his book looking for *r* words until he utters the correct one, for which he can be given some type of positive reinforcement. No mention is made of the repetitions being *stuttering.* They are simply used by you as a cueing device to help him find the correct word and thereby earn a reward. Thus, repetitive behavior becomes associated with positive instead of negative values. At the same time, the child is introduced to phonetic analysis, which may aid him in improving his reading skills. After he has found the word you have been thinking of, he can spell it orally or graphically and construct sentences with it.

In summary, therapy for the young stutterer is dependent upon the symptoms exhibited. Environmental, indirect, and the first level of direct therapy are designed primarily to keep him unaware of his disfluencies and to reduce any pressures that may increase their frequency. The second level of direct therapy acknowledges the stuttering and attempts to identify and eliminate the more gross secondary characteristics and avoidances. At all times, therapy for the young stutterer is geared to provide him with pleasant speaking experiences to reduce the sting of his frustrations. At no time should he be forced to analyze or "face" his problem.

THE ASSESSMENT OF THE OLDER STUTTERER

The older secondary stutterer generally refers to the teen-age high schooler and the adult. By this time he is usually having a great deal of difficulty in expressing himself. He exhibits struggle and tension in his oral musculature, and words are becoming mountains to be climbed. Maladaptive speech habits and the emotional reactions to them are becoming calcified. Ingrained hierarchical secondary symptoms are being learned to cope with the frustrating and sometimes panicky feeling that results when the stutterer finds himself stuck and unable to make the transition from one sound or syllable to the next. Feelings of helplessness predominate, and fears become attached to specific situations. Avoidance, escape, and release mechanisms serve to compound his difficulty and only serve to add to the bizarreness of his behavior. He is like a man who thinks he is walking through some thick mud, and the more he tries to extracate himself from his predicament, the more he finds himself in trouble. He then realizes he is in quicksand and begins to thrash around with any part of his body he thinks will help him get out only to find himself sinking deeper. Finally he gives in to fear, helplessness, and panic. When a secondary stutterer is referred to you, and particularly if he seeks you out, he is desperately in need of the kind of understanding, help, and compassion that only you, the therapist, can give him.

The Initial Interview

Stutterers will come to you with varying attitudes. Some have had a great deal of therapy and have not been helped. They may feel forlorn and defeated. Others appear more cheerful and hopeful; some claim that they do not care and are not bothered by their handicap and act as if they are doing you a favor by coming for the interview, while others expect you to utter some magical incantations and thereby cast out their stuttering devil. Whatever the attitude, you should make it clear from the outset that any gains the stutterer makes in coping with his problem will be made through his own efforts. You make it known to him that you will provide support and information that may be useful to him in learning to talk more fluently. This writer does not advocate the promise of a cure; *improvement* is considered the key word. After outlining the relationship that is to exist between you and the stutterer, a brief review of the complete plan of therapy should be provided. Goals and subgoals can be discussed, and some of the activities to accomplish them are described.

During the interview, obtain some knowledge about the type of person with whom you are dealing. Learn to listen with the third ear, that is, not only be aware of your client's stuttering behavior but also of what he is telling you about himself while he stutters. It has been said that the eyes are the windows of the soul, and nowhere does a stutterer reveal himself more than through his eyes. Sometimes they say "I am embarrassed and ashamed by the way I talk. What must you be thinking about me" as they turn away from you. Or they may be used as coping and release devices when the stutterer finds himself stuck and tries to force or squeeze out the words with them. The stutterer also reveals himself through the quality of his voice. Does he sound as if he is feeling sorry for or pitying himself? Is he saying "O God, the pain. Why me. Why was I ever born?" Does he show weakness and helplessness? Does he seem to fight and attack his difficult sounds or words as though he is angry and feeling hostile towards the whole world? All these factors need to be taken into consideration if you are to learn how to motivate your client.

To learn more about the stutterer's attitudes towards communication, it is recommended that the Erickson (1969) attitude assessment scale be given. This is a true-false scale consisting of thirty-nine items containing such statements as "I am a good mixer. I often feel nervous when talking. I am pretty confident about my speaking ability." The stutterer's replies should give you some insight into his covert life. If there is not enough time to administer this scale during the initial interview, it may be taken home to be completed.

In addition to learning about the stutterer's perceptions, you should also be making mental notes of what he is doing that is preventing him from speaking normally. It will be necessary during therapy to help him unlearn his maladaptive behaviors. Observe what he does before he attempts his difficult words, what he does once he is in process of uttering the word, and then what he does after he has completed the word. Is he hesitant in the attempt or does he approach his difficulty in a forthright manner? Once he is in the block, does he go right through it or does he back out and try again? Does he reduce the tension in his speaking apparatus or does he blast out of his blocks? Once the word is uttered, does he tend to flee from the scene of the crime or does he proceed in a relatively calm, unhurried fashion? Along with your observations, it is recommended that the Lanyon (1967) test of stuttering severity be administered. This test consists of sixty-four true-false questions and is designed to determine how well the stutterer is in contact with his own symptoms. Some of the statements are "When I cannot say a word, there are little tricks I can use to help me. I sometimes clench my teeth when I talk. I tend to make extra noises when I talk." Check your observations with those of your client in order to determine the degree of objectivity he has about his own symptoms.

Difficulty Hierarchy

During the initial and subsequent interviews, a situational difficulty hierarchy should be constructed. Brutton and Shoemaker (1967) suggest listing the situations that are communicatively unpleasant and arranging them into categories such as (1) using the telephone (2) classroom activities and (3) requesting assistance from other people. The specific situations within each category are ranked according to degree of unpleasantness, and during therapy, those containing the least amount are worked on first. For example, under the category "using the telephone," Brutton and Shoemaker listed three specific situations (1) telephoning to make an appointment (2) placing a long distance call and (3) receiving a telephone call from a friend, which would then be ranked according to degree of difficulty. If receiving a telephone call from a friend was found to generate the least amount of negative emotion, it would be first to be worked on in therapy.

To further probe the stutterer's fear, sruggle, and avoidance reactions, the Woolf (1967) inventory is recommended. Another excellent inventory is The Stutterer's Self Ratings of Reactions to Speech Situations (Johnson et al., 1963).

Further Assessment Procedures

In addition to determining the attitudes and symptomatology of the stutterer, a measure of predictability, adaptation, and consistency should be obtained. This information provides useful guidelines for structuring therapy. The predictability results tell how well the stutterer is in contact with his visceral feedback.

A stutterer who is in tune with his feelings regarding whether he will stutter on a particular word will likely have a high predictability percentage, whereas the stutterer who denies these feelings and refuses to acknowledge his problem will probably have a low score. The adaptation score will indicate whether a stutterer will quickly profit from successive exposure to difficult verbal and situational material, while the consistency index will give information regarding the conditioned strength of the stuttered response to certain verbal cues. In general, the stutterer who is highly adaptive and inconsistent in his stuttering would seem to profit more from early exposure to repetitive speaking situations, such as telephoning to various places of business seeking information, stopping people in the street to ask for directions and conducting house-to-house surveys on selected topics. In contrast, a low adapting, highly consistent stutterer would likely require more preparation as a protection against experiencing too much failure. Outside speaking assignments would have to be more highly structured, beginning with those that are relatively easy and progressing to the more difficult ones.

Predictability Percentage

It is suggested that a predictability percentage be obtained for both single words and oral reading. To calculate the percentage for single utterances, a list of twenty words is presented one at a time to the stutterer. These words should have relevance to him, such as *telephone, father, love,* and *hate.* If he seems to have more difficulty with a particular sound or sounds such as *p, t,* or *k,* words containing these sounds can be included. As a word is shown, he is to indicate whether he expects to stutter on that particular word before it is attempted. He is then instructed to "Say the word," and both his predictions and actual responses are recorded. From this data two predictability percentages are computed. The first percentage is obtained by dividing the number of actual stutterings by the number of expected stutterings. Thus, if stuttering was predicted on fifteen words, and ten of these words were actually stuttered, the predictability percentage would be $10/15 = 67$ percent. The second percentage is determined by dividing the number of words not stuttered by the number of words not expected to be stuttered. For example, if five words were predicted not to be stuttered, and four of them were actually said without stuttering, the predictability percent would be $4/5 = 80$ percent.

To determine the actual and expected stutterings from the oral reading passage, the stutterer is given a copy of the passage and instructed to read it silently and underline all the words on which he expects to stutter. Then he is given a fresh copy of the passage to read aloud, and you underline all the words that are actually stuttered on your copy. Compare the actual and expected stutterings and compute your percentages as you did for the single words.

Adaptation

To obtain the adaptation percentage, have the stutterer read a selected passage five times. Tape-record the responses and compute the relationship between the first and the fifth reading by subtracting the number of words stuttered on the fifth reading from the number of words stuttered on the first reading. Then divide the figure obtained by the number of words stuttered on the first reading. The computation is actually much easier than the explanation just provided. For example, if there were 50 stuttered words on the first reading and 10 stuttered words on the final reading, simply subtract 10 from 50 and divide by 50 ($40/50 = 80\%$). This percentage would indicate a high degree of adaptability.

Consistency

The consistency percentage is computed from the same five readings that provided the adaptation information. To calculate the consistency percentage, list all the stuttered words in the final reading of the oral passage and determine which of these were also stuttered in all previous readings. Thus, if 20 words were stuttered during the fifth reading, compare which of these words were also stuttered in the fourth, third, second, and first readings. If 15 of the 20 words fall into this category, the consistency percentage is $15/20 = 75\%$, which is considered a high level of consistency.

From the data obtained, you should have an idea of the type of individual with whom you will be working. Your opinions, of course, are only tentative and may need to be changed or modified in time, but at least you have gained some information with which to formulate a plan of therapy.

THERAPY OF THE OLDER STUTTERER

Introduction

The practicing clinician is currently being bombarded with a plethora of therapeutic rationales and techniques for the treatment of stuttering with each of their proponents claiming positive results. One wonders whether it is the adequacy of the rationales and their resultant techniques or the charisma of the therapist that helps the stutterer improve his speaking performance. No doubt the therapy you are practicing today is dependent on the philosophy of the school from which you graduated, or it is the type of therapy you have gleaned for yourself and with which you feel comfortable. Most of the clinicians I have met, however, are dissatisfied with their results and are constantly looking for ways to improve their performance. The purpose of the following pages is to introduce you to the melange of therapies in vogue in the hope that they will lead you to a more in-depth study of procedures you had not considered before and that you feel may add to your therapeutic armatorium. In the presentation of these therapies, I shall try to be as objective as possible.

Types of Therapy

The types of therapy being practiced include rhythm stimulation, shadowing, masking, delayed auditory feedback, prolonged rate, classical and operant deconditioning, air flow, and MIDVAS. As each of these therapies is subsequently described, it will be noted that they are either fluency or stuttering oriented. The fluency oriented therapies ignore the stuttering or penalize it and reward fluent production while the stuttering therapies attempt to shape and modify the stuttering with the goal of reducing its abnormality to a minimum.

Fluency Oriented Therapies

Rhythm, shadowing, delayed auditory feedback, prolonged speech, some forms of auditory masking and deconditioning, and air-flow therapies are designed to eliminate or reduce stuttering as quickly as possible and replace it with nonstuttered speech. This type of therapy is probably more appealing to many therapists and stutterers because fluency is quickly achieved, and the stutterer does not have to come to grips with and face his maladaptive behavior, which he finds extremely unpleasant. The question to be answered, however, is whether the newly acquired fluency is maintained over time. Documented data to conclusively answer this question is lacking.

If relapse over a five- or three-year or shorter period of time proves to be common, the stutterer is done an injustice. To raise his hopes that fluency now belongs to him only to find that, in the space of a few short months or years, it has been taken away from him in the form of a relapse can lead to much disappointment and unhappiness. Before the stutterer begins therapy, he has formed some type of adjustment to his speech impediment. If he quickly achieves fluency and enjoys its rewards, his former adjustment is replaced with a different set of attitudes, opinions, and ego defense mechanisms. If the new fluency is found to be too fragile under stress, the readjustment the stutterer is forced to make can be extremely painful. It would have been better not to have begun therapy than to raise false hopes and have them shattered. On the other hand, if the fluency oriented therapies prove effective, a great deal of the effort and emotional struggle a stutterer must exert to be constantly facing and working with his abnormalities can be prevented.

Stuttering Oriented Therapies

MIDVAS (see page 215) and some types of auditory masking and operant deconditioning are examples of stuttering oriented therapies. The stutterer learns to manipulate his speech and sees his stuttering as an opportunity to struggle not only for speech control but for self-control. He enters into countless situations in which he attempts to become more objective towards his oral gyrations and views his abnormal coping mechanisms with curiosity instead of fear, shame, and disgust. In addition, he analyzes, feels, and wraps himself around his stuttering before beginning to shape and modify it towards more acceptable production.

Following is a description of each of the types of therapy mentioned above. The discussion of the fluency oriented therapies will follow the format of the Ingham and Andrews (1973) article in which representative procedures will be selected and, in some cases, described in greater detail.

Rhythm

With rhythm therapy, the stutterer gains quick fluency by speaking to a pre-set rhythm. This is provided either by the use of a metronome or by having the stutterer tap out the rhythm with his finger. The syllables are all uttered evenly and rhythmically without differentiation of stress. Parameters such as pitch and loudness are reduced to a minimum. The type of speech produced sounds artificial, slow, and monotonous. Brady (1971) combines metronome and behavior therapy to provide the stutterer with a more natural prosodic pattern. First the stutterer learns to talk to a metronomic beat in a very slow and relaxed fashion. Then he obtains more normal prosody by varying his pauses and the number of words spoken to the metronomic beat. Finally he works through a hierarchy of feared situations, beginning with those containing the least fear to the most feared, with the aid of the metronome and then without. Andrews and Harris (1964) used syllable-timed speech without the aid of a metronome with children, adolescents, and adults and reported that they had their greatest success with children. They also did not use rhythm as their sole technique but combined it with group discussions.

Shadowing

This therapy rests upon the assumption that the stutterer has a defective perceptual feedback mechanism and that the missing ingredients are supplied by the auditory behavior of you, the therapist. Shadowing is analagous to choral speech whereby both you and the stutterer simultaneously read the same passage. When the stutterer achieves fluency, you begin to slowly fade out by reducing and finally eliminating your verbal contribution. When stuttering begins to return, you reenter the reading situation until fluency is again achieved. The fading out and reentering phases are performed as often as necessary until the stutterer can maintain his fluency without your aid.

Spontaneous conversation may also be used in which you begin to discourse on a selected topic. The stutterer watches the movements of your mouth and attempts to verbally shadow your utterances. In other words, he tries to say what you are saying as simultaneously as possible. Some lag time is necessarily incurred, but it becomes minimal as the stutterer practices this technique and even begins to anticipate your thoughts. A more in-depth study of other types of shadowing techniques may be found in the article by Cherry and Sayers (1956), and its effectiveness with other types of therapy is discussed by Ingham and Andrews (1973).

Delayed Sidetone and Prolonged Rate

Since Goldiamond's (1965) finding that a stutterer could beat the aversive stimulus of delayed sidetone by drastically slowing down his speech, the two concepts of delayed sidetone and prolonged speech were united. Goldiamond devised a reading rate program using delayed sidetone; however, he claimed that this type of therapy could be performed without the aid of the sidetone equipment. Curlee and Perkins (1969) modified the Goldiamond treatment by substituting conversational speech for reading and added time-out and systematic desensitization procedures. They encouraged the stutterer to engage in conversation with his therapist and to talk about any topic he wished. Their conditioning program followed two phases. In the first phase, the stutterer was taught to slow down his speaking rate by prolonging his syllables and speaking in short phrases until his utterances coincided with the delayed sidetone, which was set at 250 msec. This delay slowed the speaking rate to approximately 30-35 words per minute and generally resulted in fluency. This fluency was referred to as the 250 msec rate. The stutterer was to maintain this rate while the sidetone delay was reduced in 50 msec steps until 0 msec delay was reached. Once this had been accomplished, the delayed sidetone was set at 200 msec delay, and the stutterer's speaking rate was increased until it coincided with this delay. Then the same procedure of reducing the sidetone delay in 50 msec steps was followed as the stutterer continued to speak at the 200 msec rate. This was repeated as the sidetone delay was set at 150, 100, 50, and finally 0 msec delay, thus instating fluent speech at a normal rate.

To assist the stutterer in achieving fluency, a time-out procedure was applied whenever any stuttering was evidenced. To accomplish this, the stutterer and therapist conversed in a room lighted by a single lamp. Whenever stuttering occurred, the clinician turned the light out for 30 seconds, and the stutterer had to stop talking. At the end of the period, the light was turned on and talking was resumed. The light interval was reduced in 5-second steps when the no-stuttering criterion was achieved until a 5-second light out limit was reached. If the stuttering criterion which was set at no more than two stutterings in any 5-minute interval was exceeded, the time-out was increased to the preceding time limit until no stuttering was again achieved. That is, if the stuttering criterion was exceeded at the 15-second time-out limit, it was then increased to 20 seconds until no stuttering was evidenced. This concluded the first phase of the treatment.

The second phase was designed to wean the stutterer away from the clinical room into the everyday situations he normally encountered. These situations were arranged into a difficulty hierarchy, and the stutterer began working on his least difficult situations. He had to demonstrate the same fluency he had in the therapy room before moving on to the next level of difficulty.

Many clinicians do not have access to expensive delayed sidetone equipment. As Goldiamond (1965) stated, it is possible to train the stutterer to slow down his speaking rate without the aid of this equipment. You can teach the stutterer to drag out his sounds until fluency is reached, then slowly begin to increase his rate from this baseline, returning to a slower rate whenever stuttering is produced and repeating the procedure until the no-stuttering criterion is achieved. Rate continues to be increased until normal speech is obtained.

Masking

Introducing a loud sound into the stutterer's ears while he is communicating has been shown to dramatically reduce the frequency of his stuttering (Shane, 1955; Maraist and Hutton, 1957). This technique has been employed in therapy with varying results (Trotter and Lesch, 1967 Perkins and Curlee, 1969; and Gruber, 1971). Trotter and Lesch, and Perkins and Curlee used masking in an effort to reduce or prevent stuttering from occurring. The masking noise was introduced either when the stutterer anticipated difficulty or when he was beginning to stutter. Trotter and Lesch used a portable voice masker for two and one-half years and found its positive results to be situation specific. There was no carryover into those situations where the masker was not used. In addition, Perkins and Curlee reported some dissatisfaction with the aid. The three stutterers who used the masker stated that it was not effective during telephone conversations since an ear plug had to be removed, thereby eliminating the masking noise and its effect. One stutterer reported he felt success with the masker because it made him feel alone and isolated even though he was in a social situation. Since he did not stutter when he was actually alone, he also did not stutter in situations where he had the same feeling. The subjects felt the use of a voice masker was an inconvenience, inducing a hearing loss in social situations, and they feared that it could become a crutch.

Gruber (1971) did not have his stutterers turn on the masker when they anticipated the block. He encouraged them to have the block, and only when they felt themselves struggling were they to turn on the masker. The prime purpose of the masker was to have the stutterer tactually monitor his speech and become highly aware of the feeling that occurred as his struggle reactions gave way to a smooth transition to the following sound. Thus it was used to help him modify his blocks and consciously experience a smooth pullout. To heighten their tactual sensation, the stutterers were instructed to slow down their utterance as they were pulling out of the block and to focus on the transitional movements. None of the eleven stutterers used in the study obtained stutter-free speech. As a matter of fact, the frequency of their stuttering remained as high as before; however, the severity of their blocks was considerably reduced. In many instances they felt the tremors in their oral apparatus stop and found themselves, sometimes surprisingly, pulling out of their block. Most of the stutterers reacted positively to the masker; however, some did not want to use it because they felt it would turn into a crutch or because the noise bothered them.

Classical and Operant Conditioning

At the beginning of this section, I stated that I would try to be as objective as possible to the different types of therapy; however, I find it necessary to include a subjective statement at this point. Sometimes, in therapy and in research, painful stimuli such as electric shock and loud sounds have been inflicted upon the stutterer to reduce or study stuttering behavior. I do not intend to discuss this aspect of behavior therapy. Van Riper (1975) stated that clinicians reveal their self-concepts in the type of therapy they practice. It is my opinion that those therapists and researchers who employ painful stimuli to reduce stuttering are satisfying their own sadistic impulses. I find it difficult to understand how one individual can watch another flinch time after time. There is ample evidence that physical punishment does not eliminate but simply represses maladaptive behavior, generates anger, and produces other unhealthy side effects; yet it is continued to be used with impunity towards the stutterer. Under the disguise of theoretical models and modern sophistication, we persist in returning to the cruelty of the Middle Ages. The stutterer has enough of a negative emotional load to carry without the therapist generating more. I suggest that every time a painful shock is administered to a stutterer, the therapist or researcher administer one to himself. I positively guarantee that a significant reduction in punishment oriented therapy would occur. There is enough anger and hostility in the world without the profession of Speech and Language Pathology contributing to its supply.

In discussing the conditioning procedures, the two-factor theory of Brutton and Shoemaker (1967) and Webster and Brutton (1974) with the operant procedures of Mowrer (1971) and Ryan (1971) have been selected as representative of this type of therapy. Brutton and Shoemaker's two-factor theory accounts for the onset and development of the overt and covert aspects of stuttering by contending that the onset of stuttering, which consists primarily of the type of nonfluency often referred to as primary stuttering, occurs because of classically conditioned negative emotion such as fear and anxiety; the resultant coping behaviors, generally referred to as secondary characteristics, increase in severity over time and are acquired by means of instrumental conditioning.

In attempting to change the stutterer's emotional attitudes towards talking, the classical deconditioning procedures of desensitization, counter-conditioning, and weakened stimuli are employed. Instrumental conditioning procedures such as nonreinforcement and rewarding of an alternate response are used to modify secondary characteristics such as eye blinks and verbal behaviors such as interjections and hard contacts. Excellent definitions and the application of the concepts mentioned above are to be found in the writings of Webster and Brutton (1974). A summary of these concepts will be provided after the following section.

Before attempting to modify a stutterer's emotional attitudes and speech behavior, Brutton and Shoemaker (1967) suggest that his difficult situations be arranged on a fear hierarchy ranging from the least to the most feared. They further recommend that the situations be grouped into categories, such as telephoning, speaking to strangers, home, school, and work, with a hierarchy set up for each category. Once those situations containing the least amount of fear have been selected, the treatment begins. Working on shaping emotional attitudes and speech performance need not be mutually exclusive but may be done concurrently. As mentioned above, desensitization, counter-conditioning, and weakened stimuli or any combination thereof are used to modify emotional attitudes. In desensitization, the feared situation is presented over and over again without the unpleasant unconditional stimulus being present. Thus, if speaking on the telephone is feared, the stutterer does a great deal of talking on the telephone. As much as possible, the therapist structures the situation so that no aversive consequences will result, particularly at the initiation of therapy or until the stutterer has acquired a tough skin. Counter-conditioning is similar to desensitization with the exception that the difficult situation is presented within the context of positive behaviors such as eating or relaxation. Imagination therapy may be used whereby the stutterer is first relaxed and then verbally presented with the feared situation. Weakened stimuli can be co-joined with either desensitization or counterconditioning and simply refers to the presentation of the difficult situation in graded steps so that the stutterer will not or will minimally experience any negative emotion. Thus, if the stutterer fears the telephone, he might first pick up the receiver several times until he can accomplish this without any anxiety. He then moves on to the next step of dialing, then permitting the telephone at the other end to ring, and finally speaking to the person at the other end of the line.

In reducing a stutterer's coping behaviors, Brutton and Shoemaker (1967) suggest nonreinforcement or massed practice. In this procedure, the stutterer selects a characteristic such as an eye blink and repeats this performance over and over again before or during the utterance of words upon which he does not expect any difficulty, under the assumption that he will ultimately fatigue this response. After he has practiced this behavior in therapy, he is to immediately enter into an outside social situation and attempt to communicate without using his eye blinks. Another method of eliminating coping behaviors is to reward an alternate response. The stutterer is praised for any variation he can achieve in his eye blinks. Records can be kept of the number of instances he was able to stutter without eye blinks, or when he took on a feared situation for the first time, or when he reduced some of his characteristic avoidance and postponement techniques.

Mowrer (1971) and Ryan (1971) use operant conditioning procedures to alleviate stuttering in both children and adults.

Their therapy design is to increase the utterances of the stutterer from unstructured single words to structured single words, two words, and three-word phrases, and ultimately to lengthy, connected discourses. Base rates are determined and criteria are established, which the stutterer must reach before he can continue to the next level of verbal complexity. Criteria levels generally consist of no more than one stutter for every two minutes of talking. Rewards are provided for fluent utterances. Mowrer states that social praise such as "Good" accompanied by a smile, a head nod, and eye contact was effective with high school children and adults, particularly when provided by peers. For elementary and junior high school students, money was more effective. Stuttering was not permitted. If it occurred, it was punished by the verbal command stop, or if money was used, the child would lose a portion of his earnings. Provision was made for transfer and maintenance after fluency had been established. During the transfer phase, the therapist worked with the stutterer providing encouragement and support as he attempted to use his fluent speech in a number of social situations in his natural environmental settings. During the maintenance phase, the therapist continued to support the stutterer but began to reduce their contacts, while at the same time shifting the responsibility of monitoring his speech, by means of positive reinforcement, to important people in his environment.

Airflow

There is a belief among some speech scientists and speech pathologists that the cause of stuttering may be a malfunctioning of the peripheral neuromuscular relationships, or it may be localized no higher in the central nervous system than the lower brain stem, resulting in faulty respiratory and phonatory behavior (Baken, 1974). This hypothesis is reflected in the return of a type of therapy in which the stutterer is taught to consciously monitor his breath stream to produce a sustained laryngeal tone and smooth articulatory transitions (Schwartz, 1976). Schwartz (1975) hypothesizes that abnormal laryngeal functioning is the core of the stuttering block and is caused by excessive contraction of the posterior cricoarytenoid (PCA) muscles. Thus, the stutterer attempts to initiate phonation when his vocal folds are in a tense, open position. Schwartz claims that this laryngeal behavior is a part of the airway dilation reflex (ADR), which is automatically generated under conditions of emotional stress. This stress occurs because of the stutterer's fears of sounds, words, and situations. The stutterer's attempt to cope with his malfunctioning vocal mechanism then sets off the chain of secondary behaviors of struggle and avoidance.

Gruber (1975) contends that the core of the stuttering block occurs long before the stutterer acquires fears of words and situations and is represented primarily by the nonmorphemic repetitions of sounds and syllables and prolongations. Bloodstein (1975) states that stuttering does not become cued into specific words and situations until the third phase is reached and that fears do not enter the picture until the fourth or final phase. Gruber further contends that respiratory and phonatory abnormalities are coping behaviors and are part of the "obstacle reflex" that the stutterer automatically generates to try to stop the annoying repetitions and prolongations. He hypothesizes that the "obstacle reflex" consists of the following behaviors occurring either successively or simultaneously: adduction of the vocal folds, tension of the thorax, and tension and protrusion of the abdomen thereby trapping the air and increasing tension in the speaking mechanism. This reflex is normal whenever more strength is needed to remove an obstruction such as a rock from a garden or lift a 300 lb. weight but becomes maladaptive when the stutterer tries to talk from this position. Partial support for this reflex is to be found in the articles of Van Riper (1936) and Freeman and Ushijima (1975).

Empirical evidence concerning respiratory and laryngeal malfunctioning and their interrelationships during stuttering is meager and must await further evidence before this issue is resolved. The first Hayes Martin conference, the proceedings of which were published and edited by Webster and Furst (1975), is a step in the right direction, and it is hoped that more research of the type suggested by this conference will be forthcoming. In any event, there are few therapists who would not agree that laryngeal malfunctioning is an integral component of stuttering behavior. The question arises how this behavior can be counteracted. Should it be worked with directly, indirectly, or be ignored. Schwartz (1976) has revived and modified the ancient air-voice- and movement therapy and uses conscious control of the breath stream to counteract abnormal laryngeal functioning. First the stutterer inhales and exhales normally several times until he becomes aware of the sensation of air entering and leaving his mouth. When this air consciousness has been achieved, he is trained to utter a word, with the first syllable spoken slowly and concentrating on stretching out the vowel, only after he has felt the air being expelled through his mouth. The purpose of generating air flow before verbal utterance is to insure vocal fold vibration. During the preverbal period, the stutterer does not preform the initial sound. At first he may be able to speak only one word per breath, but with practice he increases from single words to phrases until he achieves a normal rate of talking.

MIDVAS

It seems fitting that the discussion of therapy for the older stutterer should be brought to a close with the MIDVAS approach of Van Riper (1973). His therapy is primarily stuttering oriented and demands a great deal of emotional strength on the part of the stutterer and his therapist. The final word on the fluency vs. the stuttering oriented therapies has not been written, but whatever the outcome, Doctor Van Riper has had a great, if not the greatest, influence on the direction of therapeutic intervention in this century.

MIDVAS is an acronym wherein each letter stands for a separate concept and provides the clinician with therapeutic structure. The letters stand for M—Motivation, I—Identification, D—Desensitization, V—Variability, A—Approximation, and S—Stabilization. Therapy is conducted in this sequence beginning with motivation and ending with stabilization.

Motivation is a two-way process. The stutterer provides his own motivation because he is in a miserable situation. He cannot talk adequately and finds his inability to communicate a barrier to obtaining some of the better things in life. His stuttering is onerous, frustrating, and extremely undesirable, and he wants to eliminate it. You, the therapist, provide motivation by revealing yourself as a competent person who understands and offers the stutterer hope that his speech can be changed. Motivation for the stutterer begins to wane when he discovers some of the unpleasant things he has to do. When the overall plan of therapy is presented to him and he discovers that you are not going to cure him or provide him with some magic pill or perform stuttering surgery, but that he is going to have to reveal his abnormality to the world and take responsibility for his own behavior, his courage and resolve may begin to sink. It is at this point that you provide him with the support and counseling he needs. Take his stuttering into your own mouth and show him how it can be manipulated. Make a telephone call and stutter so he can see that the roof is not going to fall on his head. This could be the impetus that will propel him toward more heroic efforts on his own part. Set up minimum and maximum goals that you feel can be achieved. Reward him for both effort and accomplishment, no matter how small, that move him closer to attaining his final goal of speech that contains a minimum of abnormality.

During the identification phase, no attempt is made to modify the stuttering. This is the period of discovery when the stutterer becomes aware of the things he does that prevent him from saying his words easily. It is a time for inventory taking in which all the behaviors to be unlearned are listed. These include the struggle reactions, loci of tension, verbal and nonverbal postponement devices such as "um" or "well" or "you know," loss of eye contact, circumlocutions, and substitutions. They also include the escape devices such as squeezing the word out with his eyes or jerking his jaw, which are used to free the stutterer from his block. Difficult situations are identified, and this is a good time to set up a difficulty hierarchy. Find out which situations contain little fear and which ones have a great deal of fear. Once the inventory has been completed, you and the stutterer decide upon their order of reduction and elimination. Generally, the more gross symptoms and the easier situations will be worked with first.

The desensitization aspect of therapy is primarily designed to reduce the stutterer's negative emotional attitudes towards his own impediment. He begins to face his problem and thereby reduces some of the fear, shame, and embarrassment load he has been carrying. It is a time for working towards getting a tougher skin and viewing stuttering as a problem that contains a solution rather than as a curse that has been given to him. Many techniques to accomplish this have already been suggested in previous sections. Disinhibition, counter-conditioning, and weakened stimuli can be employed. Pseudostuttering, sometimes referred to as faking, in which the stutterer tries to imitate his real stuttering on words he feels he can say fluently, may be used. If he can take it, he is given a stuttering bath in which he is required to do a great deal of pesudostuttering. Goals can be set up to determine the number of consecutive words on which he can fake stuttering. These and many other techniques for desensitization suggest themselves to the enterprising therapist.

The two concepts of variability and approximation form the modification portion of the therapy. In the variability phase, the stutterer is taught to change his behavior to break up his stereotyped patterns. He is shown and begins to experiment with different types of stuttering. At times he may even exaggerate his symptoms or adopt other secondary behaviors. For example, if he habitually lowers his head when in a block, he may try to raise his head, or if he lowers it to the right, he may try lowering it to the left. This may seem bizarre at first, but the rationale behind this is for the stutterer to consciously have some say over his own behavior. Many stutterers insist they cannot say their difficult words without their old involuntary patterns and that the shift to more normal production is impossible for them. This method shows them in a concrete fashion that they do not have to talk in their old way but that they do have some control over their responses. When he becomes convinced that his speech can be modified, the stutterer will be ready to move towards more acceptable production.

During approximation, the stutterer moves closer to his target of fluent stuttering. To accomplish this, Van Riper (1973) relies heavily on cancellations, pullouts, and preparatory sets. In the cancellation process, the stutterer stops after he has stuttered, attempts to analyze what happened, and then tries to say the word in an easier way. During pullouts, he works towards correcting his maladaptive behavior while it is happening, thus enabling him to make a smooth transition to the following sound. A pullout may be likened to a cancellation without the pause. Preparatory sets are used when the stutterer anticipates difficulty on a particular word. He learns to initiate these words with light contacts and smooth transitions. He finds himself stuttering in an easy, fluent fashion in contrast to his old habits of struggle and tension.

Stabilization, the final stage in therapy, consists primarily of the stutterer continuing to set up assignments for himself in consultation with you, his therapist. The purpose of these assignments is to strengthen his new approaches towards feared words and situations and to help him cope with his stuttering should relapse occur. It is a weaning-away process in which your contacts with him become fewer until he becomes his own therapist. When should therapy come to an end? Van Riper (1973) claims that the stutterer will tell you when to terminate therapy. He begins to fail to show up for appointments or becomes impatient with the performance of other stutterers during group sessions and even appears bored with stuttering and himself. He loses excitement about his own fluency and takes it for granted. At this point, future encounters between you and the stutterer should be on a co-therapist basis and move in the direction of social rather than therapist-client relationship.

References

1. Andrews, G. and Harris, M.: *The Syndrome of Stuttering.* London, Heinemann, 1964.
2. Baken, R.: Overview of the conference. In *Vocal Tract Dynamics and Dysfluency,* L.M. Webster and L.C. Furst (Eds.). New York, Speech and Hearing Institute, 1975.
3. Bloodstein, O.: *A Handbook on Stuttering,* 2nd ed. Chicago, National Easter Seal Society for Crippled Children and Adults, 1975.
4. Brady, J.P.: Metronome-conditioned speech retraining for stutterers. *Behavior Therapy, 2:*129-150, 1971.
5. Brutton, G.J. and Shoemaker, D.J.: *The Modification of Stuttering.*

Englewood Cliffs, Prentice-Hall, 1967.
6. Cherry, E.C., and Sayers, B.M.: Experiments upon the total inhibition of stammering by external control and some clinical results. *J Psychosomatic Res, 1*:233-246, 1956.
7. Cooper, E.B.: Structuring therapy for therapist and stuttering child. *J Speech Hearing Dis, 30*:75-78, 1965.
8. Curlee, R.F., and Perkins, W.H.: Conversational rate control therapy for stuttering. *J Speech Hearing Dis, 34*:245-250, 1969.
9. Davis, D.M.: The relation of repetitions in the speech of young children to certain measures of language maturity and situational factors: Part 1. *J Speech Dis, 4*:303-318, 1939.
10. Egland, G.O.: *Speech and Language Problems—A Guide for the Classroom Teacher.* Englewood Cliffs, Prentice-Hall, 1970.
11. Eisenson, J. and Ogilvie, M.: *Speech Correction in the Schools,* 2nd ed. New York, Macmillan Publishing Co., 1977.
12. Erickson, R.L.: Assessing communication attitudes among stutterers. *J Speech Hearing Res, 12*:711-724, 1969.
13. Freeman, F.J. and Ushijima, T.: Laryngeal activity accompanying the moment of stuttering: A preliminary report of EMG investigations. *J Fluency Dis, 1*:36-45, 1975.
14. Goldiamond, I.: Stuttering and fluency as a manipulable operant response class. In *Research in Behavior Modification,* L. Kramer and L.P. Ullmann, (Eds.). New York, Holt, Rinehart and Winston, 1965.
15. Gruber, L.: The use of the portable voice masker in stuttering therapy. *J Speech Hearing Dis, 36*:287-289, 1971.
16. ——: Stuttering: A rationale for therapy. *WMU J Speech Therapy, 12*:13-14, 1975.
17. Ingham, R.J. and Andrews, G.: Behavior therapy and stuttering: a review. *J Speech Hearing Dis, 38*:405-441, 1973.
18. Johnson, W.: *The Onset of Stuttering.* Minneapolis, University of Minnesota Press, 1959.
19. Johnson, W., Darley, F.L., and Spriestersbach, D.C.: *Diagnostic Methods in Speech Pathology,* 2nd ed. New York, Harper and Row, 1963.
20. Johnson, W., Brown, S.F., Curtis, J.F., Edney, C.W., and Keaster, J.: *Speech Handicapped School Children,* 3rd ed. New York, Harper and Row, 1967.
21. Lanyon, R.I.: The measurement of stuttering severity. *J Speech Hearing Res, 10*:836-843, 1967.
22. Luper, H.L. and Mulder, R.L.: *Stuttering Therapy for Children.* Englewood Cliffs, Prentice-Hall, 1964.
23. Maraist, J.A. and Hutton, G.: Effects of auditory masking upon the speech of stutterers. *J Speech Hearing Dis, 22*:385-389, 1957.
24. Mowrer, D.E.: *Technical Research. Report S-1: Reduction of Stuttering Behavior.* Tempe, Arizona State University, 1971.

25. Peacher, W. and Harris, W.E.:   Speech disorders in World War II: Part VIII. Stuttering. *J Speech Dis, 11*:303-308, 1947.
26. Perkins, W.H. and Curlee, R.F.:   Clinical impressions of portable masking unit effects in stuttering. *J Speech Hearing Dis, 34*:360-362, 1969.
27. Ryan, B.P.:   Operant procedures applied to stuttering therapy for children. *J Speech Hearing Dis, 36*:264-280, 1971.
28. Sander, E.K.:   Frequency of syllable repetition and "stutterer" judgments. *J Speech Hearing Dis, 28*:19-30, 1963.
29. Schwartz, M.F.:   The core of the stuttering block. In *Vocal Tract Dynamics and Dysfluency.* L.M. Webster and L.C. Furst (Eds.). New York, Speech and Hearing Institute, 1975.
30. ———: *Stuttering Solved.* New York, J.B. Lippincott Co., 1976.
31. Shames, G.H. and Sherrick, C.E.:   Discussion of non-fluency and stuttering as operant behavior. *J Speech Hearing Dis, 28*:3-18, 1963.
32. Shane, M.L.S.:   Effect on stuttering of alteration in auditory feedback. In *Stuttering in Children and Adults,* W. Johnson (Ed.). Minneapolis, Universiy of Minnesota Press, 1955.
33. Shearer, W.M. and Williams, J.D.:   Self-Recovery from Stuttering. *J Speech Hearing Dis, 30*:288-290, 1965.
34. Sheehan, J.C. and Martyn, M.M.:   Spontaneous recovery from stuttering. *J Speech Hearing Res, 9*:121-135, 1966.
35. Trotter, W.D. and Lesch, M.M.:   Personal experience with a stutter-aid. *J Speech Hearing Dis, 32*:270-272, 1967.
36. Van Riper, C.:   Study of the thoracic breathing of stutterers during expectancy and occurrence of stuttering. *J Speech Dis, 1*:61-72, 1936.
37. ———: *Speech Correction: Principles and Methods,* 4th ed. Englewood Cliffs, Prentice-Hall, 1963.
38. ———: *The Nature of Stuttering.* Englewood Cliffs, Prentice-Hall, 1971.
39. ———: *The Treatment of Stuttering.* Englewood Cliffs, Prentice-Hall, 1973.
40. ———:   The stutterer's clinician. In *Stuttering: A second Symposium,* J Eisenson (Ed), New York, Harper and Row, 1975.
41. Webster, L.M. and Brutton, G.J.:   The modification of stuttering and associated behaviors. In *Communication Disorders: Remedial Principles and Practices,* S. Dickson (Ed). Glenview, Scott, Foresman and Co., 1974.
42. Webster, L.M., and Furst, L.C. (Eds.): *Vocal Tract Dynamics and Dysfluency.* New York, Speech and Hearing Institute, 1975.
43. Wingate, M.E.:   Evaluation and Stuttering, Part I: Speech characteristics of young children. *J Speech Hearing Dis, 27*:106-115, 1962.
44. Woolf, G.:   The assessment of stuttering as struggle avoidance and expectancy. *British Journal of Disorders of Communication, 2*:158-171, 1967.

Chapter 7

VOICE DISORDERS

MAYNARD D. FILTER

V OICE DISORDERS are found in one to two percent of the total population (Curtis and Morris, 1978) or in more than six percent of the school-age population (Pont, 1965; Baynes, 1966; Silverman and Zimmer, 1975). Disorders of the voice are noticeable deviations in phonatory (vocal fold vibration) and/or resonatory (amplification or dampening of the sounds above the vocal folds) features characterized by one or more of the following conditions:

1. The voice is considered different by listeners, and this difference causes listeners to pay more attention to the different voice than to the spoken message.
2. The difference in the voice interferes with the intelligibility of the spoken message.
3. The difference causes the speaker to react to listeners' reactions to his voice so that the speaker may be uncomfortable or dissatisfied with his speech.
4. The manner of voice production may actually cause physical damage to the vocal mechanisms.

Disorders of the voice may be classified according to etiology, location of the lesion, or according to how the voice sounds to the trained listener. This latter perceptual classification system is recommended because it involves a description of the deviant voice, and it may be applied to all voice disorders regardless of etiology or pathology. Frequently, the etiology of a voice disorder is unknown, and the specific pathology present cannot always be

221

determined by the otolaryngologist. For example, the exact nature of some growths on the vocal folds cannot be determined without a biopsy. In most instances, the otolaryngologist bases his opinion on visual observation of the vocal folds; therefore, a classification system based on pathology may be quite tenuous. In any event, the diagnosis of a pathology is a medical diagnosis; in many cases, the etiologies of voice problems are related to a variety of medical problems. For example, hoarseness may be a symptom in a multitude of diseases (Jackson and Jackson, 1937).

The perceptual classification system does not include a medical diagnosis but rather involves describing the acoustic characteristics of the voice. The use of this classification system requires training of the raters (listeners) in the identification and quantification of specific attributes of the voice, namely pitch, loudness, and quality as described by Van Riper (1939). The perceptual classification system will be discussed in detail later in this chapter.

The etiologies and pathologies of the voice have been explained and discussed elsewhere (Damsté and Lerman, 1975; Boone, 1977; Moore, 1971). It is the purpose of this chapter to discuss the identification, evaluation, and rehabilitation of individuals with voice disorders.

IDENTIFICATION

It is assumed that, for the vast majority of speech and language pathologists in clinical practice, over 90 percent of the children seen with voice disorders are referred by teachers, parents, and other professionals outside the medical profession. The only exceptions would be those speech and language pathologists employed in hospitals, medical centers, university medical schools, and private practice; these clinicians rely heavily on otolaryngologists and/or other physicians for referral. For these speech and language pathologists, often the medical diagnosis of the voice and/or other pathology has already been made. For the majority of speech clinicians, the child with a voice disorder is referred to the clinician before the child has been seen by medical personnel. The speech and language pathologist must decide which children should be seen by a physician. These problems concerning which children should be referred and which should not will be discussed after the evaluation by the speech and language pathologist is reviewed.

Any child with a "different" voice should be referred to the speech and language pathologist for an evaluation. The clinician employed in a school system should provide inservice training to school personnel to improve their abilities in identifying children with "different" voices. The school teachers and other professionals should be able to identify obvious voice problems and should be familiar with the characteristics of abnormal voices. Videotaped recordings of samples of children showing different types of abnormal and normal voices could provide illustrations that the speech and language pathologist could use for inservice training workshops. The emphasis of instruction should not be on describing specific voice disorders, but rather should be on differentiating normal and abnormal voices. It is the speech and language pathologist's responsibility to describe the voice; it is the educator's responsibility to refer any child with a "suspected" abnormal voice to the speech and language pathologist. Over-referral should not be discouraged, it is better to have every suspected voice problem checked rather than evaluating only those with obvious problems. If those with mild hoarseness were identified early, specific techniques could be implemented, which might prevent the development of more severe hoarseness, especially if the hoarseness were due to vocal abuse.

Often it is the classroom teacher or a parent who first notices that the child's voice is different. Parental education is very important, not only in identifying problems but also in the rehabilitation of children with voice disorders. For example, Filter (1978) found that, when the parents of voice-disordered children assisted in the rehabilitation process, the success of improving the voice increased.

Some children with voice disorders are identified by the speech and language pathologist through direct screening methods. The public school clinician may screen an entire segment of the school population. For example, all children eight to ten years of age may be screened because children of this age show the highest incidence of chronic hoarseness (Emge, 1975). The speech and language pathologist also screens for voice problems while s/he routinely screens for communication problems; the schedule for screening varies from school to school. The Education for All Handicapped Children Act (Public Law 94-142, 1975) allows screening of specific populations in a school as long as all children in that specific population (for example the third grade) are screened.

For screening of voice, each child may say the alphabet and count to twenty in a conversational voice; these activities can be accomplished in thirty seconds for each child. Children with abnormal voices identified through screening are scheduled for more complete evaluations by the speech and language pathologist.

EVALUATION

The responsibilities of the speech and language pathologist in the evaluation of individuals with suspected voice disorders include (1) determining if a voice disorder is present, (2) taking a complete case history including parental complaints, (3) describing the voice disorder in perceptual terms, (4) describing behaviors associated with the voice disorder, (5) determining whether the client should be referred to other professionals, and finally, after all data are available including opinions from other professionals if requested, (6) summarizing all findings and making recommendations. Each of these responsibilities will be discussed.

Difference or Disorder

The major decision is whether to put the individual in voice rehabilitation. Boone (1977) suggests a nine-point scale for rating the voice on each dimension of pitch, phonation quality, loudness, and resonance quality. Morris and Spriestersbach (1978) suggest a five-point scale for rating the severity of specific aspects or attributes of the voice. These types of equal-appearing interval rating scales were found to be efficient and reliable with trained listeners (Filter, Poynor, and Powell, 1976) when rating vocal fold tension and overall voice severity but showed poor reliability when rating pitch. The reliability of listener ratings of phonation quality, loudness, and resonance quality is unknown.

These types of ratings may have value when comparing groups of voices but add little information relative to the placement of the individual in rehabilitation. One of the first decisions the clinician must make is whether the severity of the voice deviation is great enough to place the child in direct rehabilitation sessions.

It is recommended that if a voice disorder is present, that is if the voice difference is judged to be outside normal limits, the individual should be placed in rehabilitation provided the medical and or psychological report does not indicate otherwise. Even if the voice disorder is mild in severity, the individual and his/her family should be educated about the disorder, and the individual should be taught to monitor his voice.

Unfortunately, the limits of normality of the voice cannot be objectively specified. The judgments of "normal" and "abnormal" are subjective and depend on the clinical skills of the speech and language pathologist. Normal hypernasality, periodicity, loundess, and pitch are all based on judgmental decisions that are extremely difficult to describe; the limits of normality vary from individual to individual and also vary according to age, sex, body build, and personality of the speaker.

We can measure and set arbitrary "limits of normality" for loudness and pitch by measuring their acoustic counterparts, intensity, and frequency respectively. The measurement of these physical parameters of sound requires elaborate instrumentation, which will be discussed later in this chapter. The values of intensity and fundamental frequency do not include enough information from which estimates of voice quality can be made because quality is a function of the interaction of intensity and frequency and is determined by the variety of frequencies present in a complex sound and the relative intensities of all the frequencies present in that sound.

There is no better or more efficient method of differentiating normal and abnormal voices than the perceptual evaluation by a trained listener; therefore, the speech clinician makes an educated decision about the severity of the voice deviation. If the voice is judged abnormal, further assessment procedures are warranted. These procedures will be explained in the perceptual description section below.

Case History

The purpose of the case history is to provide information that may identify factors that could contribute to the voice disorder. A description of the voice problem by the client, the client's parents, or other referring professionals should also be included in the case history. Often it is the child's parents, teacher, or family physician who first identifies the abnormal voice; therefore, it is important to obtain a description of the voice problem by the informant.

Case histories may be brief (Boone, 1977) or very elaborate (Morris and Spriestersbach, 1978). According to Boone (1977), important information about the voice disorder may be summarized under the following areas: (1) description of the problem, (2) onset and duration, (3) variation and consistency of the problem in various situations, and (4) description of daily vocal use. The case history forms found in Figures 7-1 and 7-2 are recommended for children and adults respectively. More complete case histories for individuals with voice disorders are available (D.K. Wilson, 1972; Morris and Spriestersbach, 1978).

Perceptual Description

Virtually all authorities on voice disorders agree that the acoustic characteristics of the voice may be divided into three major perceptual dimensions of pitch, loudness, and quality. There is also widespread agreement that deviations in pitch and loudness are fairly easy to identify, but deviations in quality are very difficult to quantify and describe. The two opposing philosophies on perceptual evaluations of voice disorders are (1) label and describe what is heard and (2) describe the behaviors but do not apply any labels.

Fairbanks (1960), Moore (1971), Boone (1977), and Morris and Spriestersbach (1978) provide relatively complete definitions of hoarseness, harshness, and breathiness. D.K. Wilson (1972) lists breathy, harsh, and hoarse under the heading of laryngeal tone; each dimension is rated on a seven-point scale of severity. Damsté and Lerman (1975) list breathiness, harshness, and hoarseness as functional dysphonias. Shanks and Duguay (1975) use "hoarseness" as an umbrella term including all voices that are

NAME:_____DATE:_____

PARENT'S NAME:_____

ADDRESS:_____

AGE:_____SEX: M F GRADE:_____SCHOOL_____

REFERRING CLINICIAN:_____

ADDRESS:_____

INTERVIEW INFORMANT:_____

FAMILY PHYSICIAN:_____

DESCRIPTION OF COMPLAINT:_____ _____

_____

_____

HISTORY OF PROBLEM (How long has problem existed; cause known?)

_____

_____

_____

HAS A PHYSICIAN DIAGNOSED THE PROBLEM (voice) PREVI-
OUSLY? YES NO

PHYSICIAN'S NAME:_____DIAGNOSIS:_____
                                    _____

PRESENT MEDICATION:_____

MEDICAL PROBLEMS:_____

HAS CHILD HAD HEARING TEST? YES NO
    IF YES, WHEN:_____

RESULTS:_____

HAS CHILD RECEIVED VOICE REHABILITATION? YES NO
    HOW LONG:_____

WHERE:_____BY WHOM:_____

DOES VOICE PROBLEM VARY (daily, weekly) :_____

Figure 7-1. Child case history.

Date of interview: _____

Name: _____

Address: _____

Phone: _____ Age: _

How long have you had this voice? _____

What do you think caused this voice? _____

_____

Do you think you have a problem? _____

Describe your voice problem: _____

_____

_____

Have you had any voice therapy? _____

Have you been seen by a physician concerning your voice? _____

Are you now on medication? _____

Do you smoke? _____ How much? _____

Do you drink heavily? _____

Do you consider yourself a tense person? _____

Rate yourself on tension: 1 = relaxed   7 = extremely tense: _____

Are you satisfied with your present voice? _____

Do you ever lose your voice completely? _____

Occupation:

Future occupation: _____

Phone: _____ Age: _____

Does voice change from day to day or week to week or during the day from morning to night? _____ If so, how? _____

Figure 7-2. Adult case history.

aesthetically unpleasant with some degree of air loss and/or noise.

Perkins (1971) avoids labeling the attributes of quality; instead he advocates describing the behaviors of quality under four elements: voicing, vocal constriction, vocal mode, and vocal focus. F. Wilson (1972) also avoided the use of specific terms for describing vocal quality; the Jewish Hospital Voice Profile provides a scale for rating the laryngeal cavity from (−4) open (relaxed) to (+3) closed (tense). A minus four rating represents extreme breathiness or whispering while a plus three rating represents extreme tension such as that found in spastic dysphonia. Figure 7-3 shows a voice profile adapted from the Jewish Hospital Voice Profile (F. Wilson, 1972). Moncur and Brackett (1974) also avoid labels such as "hoarse, harsh, breathy"; instead they describe the valving (closure) of the vocal folds in terms of *hypovalvular* to represent "not enough tension" and *hypervalvular* to represent "too much tension."

The following approach to the perceptual description of voice disorders is recommended; it includes the use of perceptual labels, ratings of severity, and descriptions of specific characteristics of the voice. Acoustic characteristics of the voice may be perceptually described and classified under the categories of pitch, loudness, and quality as shown in Figure 7-4. Each term will be explained.

Pitch

Scale value ratings of pitch have been found to be unreliable (Filter, Poynor, and Powell, 1976); therefore, a gross rating of either too high, normal, or too low as found on the voice profile in Figure 7-3 is recommended. Judgments of pitch must take into account the age, sex, body build of the speaker, the context of the message, and the speaking situation. Pitch variability should also be evaluated. Habitual and optimum pitch should always be routinely measured.

The client's habitual pitch may be found by having the client count to four and hold the vowel in "four." The client may also recite the alphabet or read a paragraph while the clinician matches the client's pitch on a piano, pitch pipe, or pure tone oscillator. The clinician could have a tape recording of a scale of musical notes, each note numbered or labeled in semitones. A

NAME:_____ BIRTHDATE:_____ SCHOOL_____ GRADE:____ SEX:___

How long has the problem existed?

In what situations is the voice better or worse?

Voice severity:　1　2　3　4　5　6　7

Articulation disorder:　Yes____　No____

Length of sustained "ah"_____

RESONATING CAVITY

NASALITY

HYPERNASAL

+3

+2

+1

0

−1

HYPONASAL

LARYNGEAL TENSION

tension　　　　　breathiness

1　2　3　4　5　6　7　　1　2　3　4　5　6　7

PITCH

−1　0　+1

Low　High

VOCAL RANGE

−1　0　+1

Monotone　Variable
　　　　　Pitch

LOUDNESS

−1　0　+1

Soft　Loud

COMMENTS:_____

Examiner:_____

Date:_____

Figure 7-3.　Voice profile.

PITCH
  Too high
  Too low
  Monopitch

LOUDNESS
  Too loud
  Too soft
  Monoloudness

QUALITY
  Resonatory
    Hypernasal
    Hyponasal
  Phonatory
    Breathy
    Harsh
    Hoarse
    Intermittent aphonia
    Complete aphonia
    Vocal fry

Figure 7-4. Preceptual classification.

tape recording of the client's voice on a tape loop could then be matched to this calibrated tape to determine the habitual pitch. For purposes of finding habitual pitch, a tape loop of the client's vowel in "four" is usually the best sample to obtain; a tape loop is simply the prolonged recorded vowel in "four" spliced together so that it fits exactly around the feed and take-up reels of the tape recorder. This tape loop is continuously played over and over, allowing the clinician to adjust the calibrated tape on another recorder until the client's voice matches the tone on the calibrated tape.

Optimum pitch is defined as the pitch that is produced with the least amount of effort and/or strain with the greatest amount of pleasantness. Optimum pitch may be found employing methods developed by Hahn et al. (1957) and Fairbanks (1960), summarized by Boone (1977). The total pitch range is found first, then optimum pitch is calculated by counting from the client's lowest pitch based on the following formulas:

$$\frac{\text{Range including falsetto}}{4} = N \qquad \frac{\text{Range excluding falsetto}}{3} = N$$

EXAMPLE: Range excluding falsetto $= 18 \quad \frac{18}{3} = N \quad N = 6$

Optimum pitch equals six notes up from the client's lowest note.

Boone (1977) suggests that, when finding the pitch range, the client should match his/her voice to a recorded voice of an individual of the same sex. A calibrated tape described above may also be employed to find the pitch range.

Habitual and optimum pitch should be no more than one note apart; if there is a difference of more than one note, the habitual pitch should be adjusted toward the optimum pitch. Ideally, habitual pitch should be the same as optimum pitch.

Loudness

Loudness may be rated as too loud, too soft, normal, or monoloudness (representing little variability in changes of loudness). Loudness varies with the speaking situation, the noise in the environment, and the conditions under which the individual must speak. It is almost impossible to define "normal loudness" in terms of the physical intensity of the voice in normal speaking situations. We can, however, evaluate the intensity of the voice in the laboratory by measuring in units of decibels the sound pressure level (SPL) of a voice with a sound level meter. Coleman, Mabis, and Hinson (1977) advocate measuring the complete intensity range of each client's voice and then comparing the client's range with norms; which they have provided for adults.

Excessive loudness or inadequate loudness are judgments that must be made by the speech and language pathologist, the client's teachers, and parents. It is highly desirable to evaluate the loudness of the child's voice in a variety of situations.

Quality

Quality problems may be divided into resonatory—those occurring above the vocal folds—and phonatory—those occurring at the level of the vocal folds. Resonatory problems are those associated with the valving of the velopharyngeal port. If the valve is closed when it should be open on the nasal sounds, hyponasality results. If the valve does not close properly, varying degrees of hypernasality occur. Sluggish or slow movement of the various muscles that close the velopharyngeal port may also result in assimilation nasality where vowels adjacent to nasal sounds in connected speech become nasalized.

Assimilation nasality and hyponasality are treated more as articulation problems rather than voice problems by this writer. If a child shows hyponasality and can breath through his/her nose easily, then the problem is considered functional and can be treated as misarticulations of the three nasal sounds. Assimilation nasality may result in nasalized vowels only in words that also include nasal sounds; in running connected speech, however, the hypernasality may spread to vowels and diphthongs adjacent to nasals even if the nasals are in separate words. For example, in the sentence "Come on over," nasality may be present in the first three vowels because of their proximity to the nasals.

Hypernasality is by far the most frequently occurring resonatory voice disorder. The hypernasality scale in Figure 7-3 shows three values from +1 to +3. The following rating scale, which is more descriptive than quantitative, has shown excellent reliability when used by graduate students in class.

0 = normal nasality
1 = mild hypernasality on vowels only
2 = obvious, noticeable hypernasality on vowels only
3 = mild hypernasality on vowels and consonants
4 = obvious, noticeable hypernasality on vowels and consonants

With ratings of 1 and 2 on the above scale, intelligibility is usually not noticeably affected; with ratings of 3, the consonants become slightly distorted, and with ratings of 4, intelligibility is significantly affected with noticeable imprecise production of most consonants along with hypernasality on virtually all vowels and diphthongs. The above scale limits the range of rated hypernasality of vowels to a two-point scale—"mild" and "obvious/noticeable." Morris and Spriestersbach (1978) differentiate between hypernasality (occurring primarily during vowel production) and nasal emission (occurring primarily during consonant production). It should be noted that hypernasality and nasal emission as defined above may occur simultaneously in the same utterance and could be rated separately or together as illustrated by the ratings of 3 and 4 from the above scale.

The severity of hypernasality depends on many factors including how obvious, irritating, distracting, and noticeable the hypernasality is to listeners. One of the reasons why there may be poor agreement among listeners when rating hypernasality is that each listener may have a different tolerance for hypernasality and different standards for normal and abnormal hypernasality. Perhaps in the near future we will not have to rely on listener judgments as much as we do now if methods such as computerized measurement of hypernasality as described by Lindblom, Lubker, and Pauli (1977) are used more fully. However, until the clinician has access to computers and other sophisticated laboratory equipment, we will have to depend on the clinician's trained listening.

Also in the near future, we should know more about velopharyngeal closure, the muscles involved, and the different degrees of hypernasality resulting from various degrees of incomplete closure. Research employing the EMG transducer described by Watkin, Minifie, and Kennedy (1978) should provide valuable information about the role of various pharyngeal muscles associated with closure of the velopharyngeal port. Eventually this information should lead to the development of techniques that will aid the clinician in the evaluation of behaviors associated with the production of hypernasality.

It should be noted that ratings of hypernasality are based on perceptual evaluations of the amount and severity of nasal resonance and/or nasal emission present in the speech. These ratings do not take into account the effects of the hypernasality on the speaker; an individual with a rating of two (obvious, noticeable hypernasality on vowels) might suffer socially because of the hypernasality. Blood and Hyman (1977) found that children responded negatively to other children with severe hypernasality. Their results suggest that a child with a rating of two definitely has a voice disorder and should receive appropriate treatment as soon as possible.

Phonatory voice disorders may be described employing the perceptual terms of breathiness, harshness, hoarseness, aphonia, and vocal fry.

Breathiness: Breathiness is characterized by air escaping between the vocal folds because of less than optimum approximation of the vocal folds during phonation. The severity of breathiness may vary on a continuum from a soft voice of relatively low intensity to a voice that is completely aphonic.

Harshness: Harshness is characterized by a low-pitched, tense, tight, forced voice. Overadducted vocal folds, excessive tension in the larynx and pharynx, excessive effort and force, and the frequent use of hard glottal attacks produce harshness (Boone, 1977; Filter, 1977; Morris and Spriestersbach, 1978). The harsh voice sounds rough, hard, grating; a closed mandible, tongue retraction toward the pharynx, hypercontraction of the pharynx, general hypertonicity, and excessive loudness may all be present in an individual with a harsh voice (Boone, 1977).

Hoarseness: Most authorities believe that hoarseness includes elements of both harshness and breathiness in the form of excessive tension plus incomplete closure of the vocal folds. There is still much confusion between "hoarseness" and "harshness." Hoarseness may be described as breathiness with tension (Filter, 1977). May loud hoarseness be labelled "harshness?" Morris and Spriestersbach (1978) mention "roughness" as a possible substitute for "hoarseness"; however, is not the harsh voice also rough?

Perhaps hoarseness and harshness could be differentiated on the basis of judgments of pitch, loudness, and breathiness with hoarseness showing less loudness, more breathiness, and a higher pitch than harshness. The argument could be settled by operationally defining loud, low-pitched hoarseness as "harshness" and defining all other tense, aperiodic, breathy voices as "hoarse." If in doubt, the clinician may describe the voice in other terms such as "aperiodic, low-pitched, intermittently aphonic, tense, loud." Many voices require more than one descriptive term; the more specific the description, the better.

Intermittent aphonia: This refers to a partial loss of phonation; the voice seems to come and go periodically within a word, phrase, or sentence.

COMPLETE APHONIA: Aphonia means that there is no voice, no vocal fold vibration, whispering; this condition is rare and almost nonexistent in children.

VOCAL FRY: Fry is characterized by an extremely low-pitched "popping-cracking" sound with very low rate of air flow (Mc Glone, 1967; D.K. Wilson, (1972). Reduced air flow, weak intensity, and low pitch indicate a reduction of tension in the vocal folds with the folds being thicker and more relaxed. Vocal fry may be considered a separate register or mode of producing voice (Hollien et al., 1966) and should not be considered abnormal unless it is used excessively (D.K. Wilson, 1972). We cannot measure degrees of severity of vocal fry, but we can measure the percentage of time it is present in samples of speech. Excessive use of vocal fry will result in a voice with low intensity, thus decreasing intelligibility and increasing the overall distractibility of the voice/speech message.

The major dimensions of hypernasality, harshness, hoarseness, and breathiness can be rated on equal-appearing interval scales, as suggested in Figure 7-3 for the characteristics of tension and severity. Morris and Spriestersbach (1978) suggest a 5-point scale for rating the severity of specific aspects of the voice. In a study of children with chronic hoarseness by Filter, Poynor, and Powell (1976), test-retest reliability of trained graduate student ratings of severity of hoarseness averaged .97 employing a 7-point rating scale; test-retest reliability of ratings of tension in the vocal folds averaged .90. These correlation coefficients indicate that trained listeners can indeed reliably rate specific attributes of the voice. Morris and Spriestersbach (1978) recommend that the clinician develop a training tape to periodically "calibrate" listening skills used when rating specific attributes of the voice.

Associated Behaviors

There are a variety of behaviors associated with the production of voice; some may be measured objectively, others have to be observed, others have to be rated on the basis of symptoms that are indicative of these behaviors. Figure 7-5 shows 12 associated behaviors that can be rated on a 7-point scale and/or may also be measured directly, the results of which may be summarized under

		Unsatisfactory					*Satisfactory*	
1.	Breathing Comments:	1	2	3	4	5	6	7
2.	Muscular Tension 1 tense 7 relaxed Comments:	1	2	3	4	5	6	7
3.	Ability to Carry a Tune Comments:	1	2	3	4	5	6	7
4.	Articulation Comments:	1	2	3	4	5	6	7
5.	Pitch Discrimina- tion Comments:	1	2	3	4	5	6	7
6.	Pitch Variability Comments:	1	2	3	4	5	6	7
7.	Ability to Imitate Pitch Comments:	1	2	3	4	5	6	7
8.	Loudness Variability Comments:	1	2	3	4	5	6	7
9.	Rate Comments:	1	2	3	4	5	6	7
10.	Prosody Comments:	1	2	3	4	5	6	7
11.	Self-Rating of Tension 1 extremely tense 7 relaxed Comments:	1	2	3	4	5	6	7
12.	Signs of Anxiety 1 none 7 many Comments:	1	2	3	4	5	6	7

Figure 7-5. Associated behaviors.

comments for each dimension. Following are brief comments on each behavior.

BREATHING. Does the child have adequate breath support for speech and voice? Is the child using a relaxed, appropriate method of inhalation? Is the child showing shallow breathing, rapid breathing, exaggerated respiratory movements, excessive tension in the thoracic or abdominal areas, poor posture, mouth breathing, or is the child talking too long on one breath? An excellent discussion of breathing and voice has been provided by Bloomer (1975).

MUSCULAR TENSION. The clinician may observe any obvious muscular tension, especially in the shoulders, neck, and face when the client is breathing, speaking, and producing prolonged vowels.

ABILITY TO CARRY A TUNE. The clinician may ask the client to hum a popular song or a classic such as "Yankee Doodle," or the client may actually sing a song.

ARTICULATION. This may be rated by observing the production of speech sounds in connected speech while the client is reading or speaking spontaneously. A standard articulation test may be administered if any errors are noted.

PITCH DISCRIMINATION. The client is asked which of two tones is higher, or if two tones are the same, or if the inflection of two tones raised or lowered. Stimuli for this task may be tape-recorded tones, tones from a pure tone oscillator, recordings of voices, or live voice hummed by the clinician.

PITCH VARIABILITY. The variability of pitch changes during connected speech may be rated, with a rating of 1 representing a monotone and a 7 representing overdramatic variability.

IMITATION OF PITCH. The client is asked to match the stimulus pitch by humming or singing a vowel. Stimuli may be tape-recorded or produced live. This task requires good pitch discrimination abilities on the part of the clinician.

LOUDNESS VARIABILITY. Loudness variability may be rated from "one" representing monoloudness to "seven," which represents exaggerated changes in loudness. The clinician should also listen for appropriate loudness on stressed syllables.

RATE. Unsatisfactory rate would either be too slow or too fast;

appropriate rate would be rated a seven. Fluency and speed both affect rate.

PROSODY. Prosody refers to the melody of speech including changes in pitch and loudness from syllable to syllable within words and phrases. Appropriate stress, emphasis, phrasing, and pausing all are included in ratings of prosody.

SELF-RATINGS OF TENSION. Tension may be in the form of psychological tension caused by anxiety or may be actual physical tension associated with physiological factors. It should be noted that psychological tension can cause physical tension; the two are not dichotomous. It is difficult, if not impossible, to separate "emotional" from "physical" tension; therefore the clinician should ask the client if he considers himself a tense person, and then instruct the client to rate himself on tension using a rating of 1 for very relaxed and a rating of 7 for very tense.

SIGNS OF ANXIETY. Visible anxiety may be rated from a rating of 7 representing no visible signs to a rating of 1 representing obvious symptoms present. Symptoms of anxiety include postural tension, wringing the hands, excessive perspiration, poor eye contact, inability to sit still, and other behaviors indicating the client is uncomfortable.

The following associated behaviors or evaluative procedures should also be considered with most individuals with voice disorders.

PHONATION TIME. The maximum phonation time for vowels /a/, /i/, and /u/ at constant pitch and loudness levels may be measured. Average times for girls between 8 and 17 years of age should range from 8 to 13 seconds; boys' times should average 11 to 17 seconds (D.K. Wilson, 1972). Fifteen university students in this writer's class could all phonate /a/ for more than 20 seconds; phonation times of less than 20 seconds for adults would be less than average.

LOUDNESS RANGE. The range of intensity of the voice from the softest to the loudest phonation can be easily measured with a sound level meter placed 6 inches from the speakers lips. Coleman, Mabis, and Hinson (1977) found that average intensity ranges for males was 54.8 decibels and for females 51 decibels; these were average intensity levels for their complete range of frequencies. Coleman, Mabis, and Hinson suggest that these measures should be taken before and after therapy to obtain an objective measure of improvement.

PITCH RANGE. Habitual pitch, optimum pitch, and pitch range can be given objective numerical values by measuring the fundamental frequency of the voice at different pitch levels. The pitch of the voice may be matched to a pitch pipe or pure tone oscillator, or more sophisticated procedures using a frequency counter (Coleman, Mabis, and Hinson, 1977) may be used. D.K. Wilson (1972) provides pitch charts for boys and girls from ages 1 to 18; adult males have an average fundamental frequency of 125 Hz with acceptable limits of 100–155 Hz. Adult females show an average fundamental frequency of 205 Hz with acceptable limits of 175–245 Hz. Coleman, Mabis, and Hinson (1977) found that adults have an average frequency range of 37 semitones of approximately three octaves.

ORAL PRESSURE. The ability to build pressure in the oral cavity for the production of consonant sounds is dependent on the competence of the velopharyngeal port. Various blowing exercises such as blowing up a toy balloon with the nares open and again with the nares occluded might give an indication of the competence of the velopharyngeal port; however, the clinician must make sure the child is not raising the back of the tongue to the velum and then using only air trapped in the oral cavity for blowing. A spirometer may also be used to measure the amount of air produced with nares open and occluded.

An oral manometer (Morris, 1966) is designed specifically to measure oral air pressure. With the bleed valve of the oral manometer open, the individual must exert continuous pressure, which can be read on a needle gauge. The relative pressure (bleed valve is open; therefore, pressure is not absolute) with nares open is compared with the pressure obtained with the nares occluded. If there is good velopharyngeal competence, the ratio of pressure with nares open and nares occluded will equal one.

Oral pressure measures do not correlate perfectly with measures of hypernasality or articulation competence. Dickson, Barron, and McGlone (1978) found that, in cleft palate speech, oral-nasal airflow during speaking activities differs from that produced for single vowel or blowing activities. To date, however, oral manometer pressure measures provide the most efficient methods for obtaining information about oral airflow abilities (Spriestersbach, Morris, and Darley, 1978).

Vocal Abuse

Vocal abuse may be observed and rated by teachers, parents, and the speech clinician. D.K. Wilson (1972) lists eleven common examples of vocal abuse including excessive talking, throat clearing, and coughing, with a rating of the amount and degree of each. The clinician can also observe any tension in the area of the throat and neck when the client is speaking. The clinician may actually feel the throat area to see if the client is raising the larynx during phonation, thus creating unnecessary tension.

ORAL EXAMINATION. Since the vocal folds and the internal structures and movements of the larynx cannot be observed easily, the speech and language pathologist must rely on the physician's report of the structure and function of the larynx. The speech clinician, however, can observe the structure and some functions of the velopharyngeal valve. The relative size, shape, length, and width of the hard palate, soft palate, and uvula can be observed. Movement of the soft palate during the production of /a/, /g/, and /ŋ/ and movement during a gag may be recorded. Movement of the lateral pharyngeal walls during phonation of /a/ may also be observed and described. Any constriction of the nares during phonation or blowing may also be noted.

HEARING EVALUATION. Because of the high incidence of upper respiratory infections among children with cleft palates, a hearing evaluation with this population is a must. Children with loudness deviations of the voice should also have thorough pure tone and impedance tests because a sensorineural hearing loss might cause the child to talk too loudly, whereas a conductive hearing loss might cause the child to speak too softly.

Referral to Other Professionals

The three allied professionals to whom children with voice disorders are most often referred are the audiologist, psychologist, and otolaryngologist. If the child shows a hearing loss by pure tone audiometry, he/she should be referred to the audiologist for impedance and speech audiometry. If the child shows signs of emotional problems that might contribute to the voice problem, or if the voice problem is of suspected psychogenic causes, a referral to a psychologist is necessary. For those clinicians employed in school systems, a referral to the school psychologist is the appropriate course of action. The school psychologist may then refer the child to other professionals, such as the clinical psychologist or the psychiatrist. Psychogenic voice disorders among children are rare; however, tension and anxiety among children with phonatory voice disorders may not be uncommon (Brandell and Filter, 1973). It is the psychologist's responsibility to identify, describe, and recommend management procedures for any behaviors contributing to the anxieties and tensions; therefore, for any child showing obvious signs of anxiety and/or emotional tension, a referral to the psychologist is necessary.

A referral to the otolaryngologist is necessary whenever an organic problem is suspected. The purpose of the referral to the otolaryngologist is to obtain the otolaryngologist's opinion about the structure and function of the vocal folds and about any medical problems that might be contributing to the voice disorder. The speech and language pathologist also needs to know if the otolaryngologist recommended any medical treatment. The otolaryngologist may recommend voice rehabilitation; however, the recommendation for voice rehabilitation should be made only by the speech and language pathologist after data from all professionals are in. The speech clinician makes recommendations about voice rehabilitation after reviewing information from the physician's report. The speech clinician should not ask the otolaryngologist for "clearance" or permission to begin voice therapy, but rather should ask for information about the voice disorder (Morris and Spriestersbach, 1978).

Some voice disorders show specific diagnostic behaviors, which indicate that the disorder is usually not associated with any medical problem. The following disorders do not require a referral to the otolaryngologist because the problems are considered functional in nature.

HABITUAL LOUDNESS PROBLEMS. If no hearing loss is present

and the child can imitate a voice of normal loudness during the diagnostic evaluation, the loudness difference may be considered a habit. There is a variety of factors that might cause a child to speak too softly or loudly; among the more common causes are shyness, aggressiveness, a noisy environment, sibling rivalry, and imitation of an authority figure.

HABITUAL PITCH DEVIATIONS. A child may be in the habit of using an abnormal pitch because of imitation, screaming, over-excitement, or because the abnormal pitch sounds and feels right within the child's own servosystem. If the child can imitate an appropriate pitch and has an adequate pitch range, then the child can be trained to change the habitual pitch so that eventually it matches optimum pitch.

FUNCTIONAL HYPONASALITY. If the child can close the mouth and breathe through the nose easily and imitate the /m/ sound, the hyponasality can be considered functional and may be treated as an articulation problem involving the three nasal consonants.

HABITUAL HYPERNASALITY. If the child can imitate normal voice resonance on isolated vowels and if there is good velopharyngeal movement, the hypernasality may be considered habitual as long as it is not assimilation nasality and/or nasality associated with slow, sluggish movement of the velum.

HABITUAL BREATHINESS AND/OR GLOTTAL FRY. If a normal voice quality can be produced upon imitation and/or by increasing tension, pressure, and air volume slightly, the breathiness and/or glottal fry may be considered habitual.

HABITUAL HARSHNESS. If the child can produce a voice of normal quality in vowels or a hum by decreasing tension, pressure, air volume and loudness, the harshness may be considered habitual.

All of the above habitual problems may be considered functional if a normal or near-normal voice can be produced during the diagnostic evaluation. If various procedures such as easy humming, increasing and decreasing air flow, tension, pitch, and loudness do not result in a change in the voice resulting in the voice beginning to approximate a normal voice, then the individual should be referred to the otolaryngologist. In almost all cases, a hoarse voice should be referred to an otolaryngologist except where the hoarseness is transitory and associated with the common cold. If, however, with or without a concommitant cold, the hoarseness persists for a period of time exceeding three weeks, the child should be seen by a physician.

When referring a child to the otolaryngologist, a physician's check sheet such as the one shown in Figure 7-6 may be sent to the otolaryngologist with a cover letter containing a brief description of the background, the chief complaint, and a concise summary of the speech clinician's description of the voice. It is also appropriate to mention in the cover letter that recommendations regarding a voice rehabilitation program will not be made until data are received from all consultants.

Summary and Recommendations

After reviewing all available data from the audiologist, psychologist, and medical personnel, the speech clinician recommends

---

Client's Name_____ Referred by:_____

Address:_____ Address:_____

_____

Chief Client Complaint:_____

Speech and Language Pathologist's Description of Voice:_____

Medical:

Hard Palate Structure: Appears ___normal ___abnormal

Comments:

Soft Palate Structure: Appears ___normal ___abnormal

Comments:

Nasal Cavities Structure: Appears ___normal ___abnormal

Larynx, excluding true vocal folds Appears ___normal ___abnormal

Comments:

Vocal folds Structure: Appears ___normal ___abnormal

Comments:

Structure: Appears ___normal ___abnormal

Comments:

Medical problem (s) contributing to voice deviation:

Recommended medical management:

Name of Physician:_____

Address:_____

Figure 7-6. Physician's check sheet.

an appropriate management program of voice rehabilitation or no direct voice rehabilitation. If the client shows a nontransitory voice abnormality and if the information from the consultants does not indicate otherwise, the client is usually scheduled for voice rehabilitation sessions. It is recommended that all initial voice therapy be considered trial therapy or experimental therapy. These trial sessions should be scheduled over a specific period of time such as three half-hour sessions Monday, Wednesday, and Friday for three weeks. If the client cooperates, shows changes in vocal behaviors, is satisfied with the rehabilitation program, shows evidence of progress, and if the speech clinician believes the prognosis for further progress is good, continued rehabilitative sessions are scheduled after the trial period. Because of the individual nature of the self-monitoring tasks recommended by this writer, group sessions for individuals with voice disorders are not recommended.

REHABILITATION

Each individual with a voice problem needs a unique rehabilitative program designed especially for him/her. This program must take into consideration the contributing factors that precipitate and perpetuate the voice disorder. Since each of these factors has to be managed, it is impossible to write a general rehabilitative program that would be appropriate for all individuals with a specific type of voice disorder such as vocal fold nodules. Instead, an approach to voice rehabilitation will be discussed (Filter, 1973). This approach is applicable to all types of voice disorders because the general principles may be adjusted and modified according to the unique needs of the individual. The speech clinician should already have a wide variety of rehabilitative techniques and procedures for modifying vocal behaviors; these techniques and procedures may be used with the following approach.

Proprioceptive-Tactile-Kinesthetic Approach

The objectives of this approach are to enable the client to increase awareness and learn to monitor (self-perception/proprioceptive) tactile (touch), kinesthetic (feel) feedback so that the client can (1) understand phonation and how (s)he is phonating,

(2) modify these phonatory behaviors, and (3) replace habitual behaviors with more appropriate behaviors, which will result in the production of more acceptable characteristics of pitch, loudness, and quality. The monitoring of tactile feedback includes not only the touching of one tissue against another but also the feeling of the air stream blowing past, by, or against different tissues.

Kinesthesia is the sense through which muscular weight, position, and movement are perceived. Muscular tension, contraction, relaxation, and fatigue may be perceived through kinesthetic feedback. Every muscle has sensory receptors, which are stimulated by muscle movement and stress. By becoming aware of and paying attention to the information provided by these kinesthetic receptors, the individual can understand more fully the production of voice and can develop the ability to modify muscular actions responsible for voice production.

The PTK approach does not disregard auditory feedback but rather supplements information received through auditory sensations with information received through tactile and kinesthetic sensations. Frequently, the individual with a voice disorder may be taught to differentiate specific characteristics of the voice through auditory, tactile, and kinesthetic channels. The client must be taught how the target voice feels and sounds.

The PTK approach has four basic steps, however, a concommitant activity, which is an ongoing process throughout the entire rehabilitative program, is the education of the client and parents. Education starts during the diagnostic evaluation. The procedures and results of the speech pathologist's diagnostic evaluation must be explained. If a voice pathology is found by the otolaryngologist, the otolaryngologist should explain the etiology and alternative treatment programs available. The speech clinician may also explain the information found in the physician's report. Liberal use of drawings, pictures, and models of the vocal mechanisms is recommended for explanation and clarification to clients and parents or other members of the family. For example, if one of the target goals is to raise the pitch, drawings of the vocal folds, pictures, or even working simulated models should be used to explain what is happening in the larynx.

The client should always be provided with a visual illustration or description of the target behavior. The client must understand what he/she is doing with his vocal mechanisms and what he/she should be doing, with the emphasis on the monitoring of these behaviors through tactile, kinesthetic, and auditory feedback. The educational component of the PTK approach cannot be overemphasized; in every stage the client must learn what (s)he is doing, what (s)he should be doing, how (s)he can do it, and what the feel and sound of the old behavior and new target behavior are. Keeping this educational component in mind, the four cumulative stages of the PTK approach are as follows:

Evaluation of Feedback

The major objective during this stage is to enable the client to be aware of the sensations provided by the auditory, tactile, and kinesthetic receptors during phonation. Particular attention is directed toward pressure, tension, effort, and movement of laryngeal, pharyngeal, oral, thoracic, and abdominal areas. Breathing patterns, imitating phonation on vowels and consonants, sustaining phonation, changing pitch, loudness, tensions, and specific articulatory and/or resonatory behaviors must be analyzed. For example, if the individual exhibits hypernasality, the following behaviors have to be analyzed through PTK feedback: oral opening during speech, height of tongue, retraction of tongue, tension of the jaw, tension in the velum, tension in pharyngeal walls, tension in neck muscles, movements of the larynx during phonation, sensations of air passing through the nasal and oral cavities.

Evaluation of feedback is a continuous process; the ability of the individual to monitor feedback determines the success of the rehabilitative program. The client must have a clear concept of the target and must learn to control the various sensorimotor behaviors necessary to produce the target. The next stage of the PTK approach is included with all clients showing excessive tension.

Relaxation

If there is too much tension in the laryngeal, pharyngeal, thoracic, and abdominal areas, the client must be taught to reduce and control this tension. The client must be aware of the tactile and kinesthetic sensations of tension and must be shown methods and techniques to use to reduce the tension. Basic approaches to relaxation include yawning, using a breathy sign, or a "verbal yawn," chewing, and rolling the head from side to side. Actual walking around the room and sitting in a comfortable chair with the arms dangling by the body are conducive to relaxation.

The client must become aware of the feeling of tension and relaxation in the arms, shoulders, jaw, neck, throat, chest, and velum. The clinician must also know how to relax to teach the client to do so. The scope of this chapter does not allow an in-depth discussion of relaxation techniques. An excellent explanation of relaxation may be found in Moncur and Brackett (1974).

New Phonation Patterns

The client must substitute new patterns for old. The clinician must show the child the specific target behavior and, if possible, demonstrate the behavior. The feeling of the new behavior is emphasized. For example, if the target is a breathy, relaxed hum, the client must be taught the feelings and sensations present during the production of this type of voice. This breathy hum may be learned and may be added to the breathy sigh learned during relaxation. Producing the target behavior at will 100 percent of the time should be achieved before moving on to another target behavior. Small steps should be taken along a hierarchy of behaviors. For example, the client may move from a breathy sigh to a breathy hum, to a breathy vowel, to a breathy diphthong, to a breathy vowel terminating in the /m/ sound, and so forth.

If the development of a voice with less tension is the long-range target behavior, the client may first be taught easy relaxed breathy vowels in small steps starting with a relaxed, breathy "verbal" sigh. The client is then led through a series of target behaviors progressing from relaxed, breathy voice production to a voice with normal tension and from an easy, automatic response to a task that is more socially-emotionally difficult. The chart in Figure 7-7 developed by Stone and Casteel (1974) shows a hierarchy from least to greatest likelihood of a hyperfunctional response and from least to greatest degree of muscular activity; tasks are accomplished from left to right with tasks at the bottom of the column completed first and then working up the column. The emphasis should be on improving the client's ability to monitor tactile and kinesthetic feedback while developing new phonatory patterns.

Stabilization

The new phonatory patterns are gradually practiced in a variety of situations with the clinician and are used increasingly outside the rehabilitation sessions until they become automatic and habitual. The long-range goal of rehabilitation is to enable the client to produce as nearly normal a voice as physical and

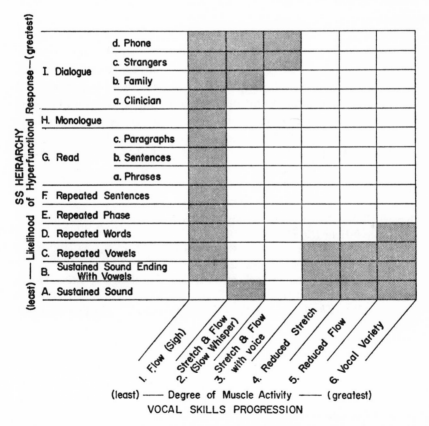

Figure 7-7. Task-response hierarchy.

psychological factors will permit. Stabilization of target behaviors is not achieved easily or quickly. Discrimination of tactile and kinesthetic sensations is usually learned slowly because voice behaviors are usually vague and abstract. Effort, tensions, movements, and pressure cannot be heard, nor can the clinician always show the client these features; instead, the client must learn to feel the PTK features while producing voice. The PTK approach should be used as a supplement to the traditional auditory, ear training, auditory discrimination approaches. Research by Haskell and Baken (1978) has shown that a client's perception of pitch during live judgments (while speaking) may differ from his perception of his pitch while listening to tape recordings of his voice. These differences in perception may be a function of the listening activity of using only the auditory channel (air conduction) while listening to tape recordings versus the listening task of using both the air conduction and bone conduction channel when listening to the voice live. These differences in perception may partially explain why many clients cannot imitate the "voice" of the clinician and may suggest that an overemphasis on auditory feedback may result in client confusions and misperceptions; training the client in the perception of tactile and kinesthetic feedback might help sort out some of this "auditory confusion."

References

Baynes, R.A.: "An incidence study of chronic hoarseness among children." *J Speech Hear Dis, 31*:172-176, 1966.

Blood, G.W. and Hyman, M.: "'Children's perception of nasal resonance." *J Speech Hear Dis, 42*:446-448, 1977.

Bloomer, H.H.: "Another look at voice and breathing." *J Mich Speech Hear Assoc, 11*:196-201, 1975.

Boone, D.R.: *The Voice and Voice Therapy,* second ed. Englewood Cliffs, P-H, 1977.

Brandell, M.E. and Filter, M.D.: "Anxiety symptoms in children with phonatory voice disorders as reported by parents." *The Division for Children with Communication Disorders Bulletin, 11*:21-24, 1973.

Coleman, R.F., Mabis, J.H., and Hinson, J.K.: "Fundamental frequency—sound pressure level profiles of adult male and female voices." *J Speech Hear Res,* 20:197-204, 1977.

Curtis, J.F. and Morris, H.L.: Disorders of voice. In Curtis, J.F. (Ed.):

Processes and Disorders of Human Communication. New York, Harper and Row, 1978.

Damste, P.H. and Lerman, J.W.: *An Introduction to Voice Pathology.* Springfield, Thomas, 1975.

Dickson, S., Barron, S., and McGlone, R.: "'Aerodynamic studies of cleft-palate speech." *J Speech Hear Dis, 43:*160-167, 1978.

Emge, M.E.: *A Longitudinal Report of Chronic Hoarseness in School-Age Children.* A paper presented at the annual meeting of the American Speech and Hearing Association, Washington, D.C., 1975.

Fairbanks, G.: *Voice and Articulation Drillbook.* New York, Harper and Brothers, 1960.

Filter, M.D.: *Communication Disorders: A Handbook for Educators.* Springfield, Thomas, 1977.

Filter, M.D.: "Parent involvement in voice rehabilitation." *J Speech Hear Assoc of Virginia, 19:*16-22, 1978.

Filter, M.D.: "Proprioceptive-Tactile-Kinesthetic feedback in voice therapy." *Lang Speech Hear Services in Schools, 5:*149-152, 1974.

Filter, M.D., Poynor, R.E., and Powell, R.L.: *A Longitudinal Study of Children with Chronic Hoarseness.* A paper presented at the annual meeting of the American Speech and Hearing Association, Houston, 1976.

Hahn, E., Lomas, C.W., Hargis, D.E., and Vandraegen, D.: *Basic Voice Training for Speech.* New York, McGraw-Hill, 1957.

Haskell, J.A. and Baken, R.J.: "Self-perception of speaking pitch levels," *J Speech Hear Dis, 43:*3-8, 1978.

Hollien, H., Moore, P., Wendahl, R., and Michel, J.: "On the nature of vocal fry." *J Speech Hear Res, 9:*245-247, 1966.

Jackson, C. and Jackson, C.L.: *The Larynx and Its Diseases.* Philadelphia, Saunders, 1937.

Lindbolm, B.E.F., Lubker, J.F., and Pauli, S.: "An acoustic-perceptual method for the quantitative evaluation of hypernasality." *J Speech Hear Res, 20:*485-496, 1977.

McGlone, R.E.: "Air flow during vocal fry phonation." *J Speech Hear Res, 10:*299-304, 1967.

Moncur, J.P. and Brackett, I.P.: *Modifying Vocal Behavior.* New York, Harper and Row, 1974.

Moore, G.P.: *Organic Voice Disorders.* Englewood Cliffs, P-H, 1971.

Morris, H.L.: "The oral manometer as a diagnostic tool in clinical speech pathology." *J Speech Hear Dis, 31:*362-369, 1966.

Morris, H.L. and Spriestersbach, D.C.: Appraisal of Respiration and Phonation. In Curtis, J.F. (Ed.): *Processes and Disorders of Human Communication.* New York, Harper and Row, 1978.

Perkins, W.H.: *Speech Pathology: An Applied Behavioral Science.* St. Louis, Mosby, 1971.

Pont, C.: "Hoarseness in children." *West Mich U J Speech Ther*, 2:6-8, 1965.
Public Law 94-142, Education for all Handicapped Children Act (November 29, 1975).
Shanks, J.C. and Duguay, M.: Voice Remediation and the Teaching of Alaryngeal Speech. In Dickson, S. (Ed.): *Communication Disorders: Remedial Principles and Practices*. New York, Scott F, 1974.
Silverman, E.M. and Zimmer, C.H.: "Incidence of chronic hoarseness among school-age children." *J Speech Hear Dis, 40*:211-215, 1975.
Spriestersbach, D.C., Morris, H.L., and Darley, F.L.: Examination of the speech mechanisms. In Darley, F.L. and Spiestersbach, D.C.: *Diagnostic Methods in Speech Pathology*, 2nd ed. New York, Harper and Row, 1978.
Stone, R.E. and Castell, R.L.: *Intervention for Functional Voice Disorders*. Mini-seminar presented at the annual convention of the American Speech and Hearing Association, Las Vegas, 1974.
Van Riper, C.: *Speech Correction: Principles and Methods*, 1st ed. Englewood Cliffs, P-H, 1939.
Watkin, K.L., Minifie, F.D., and Kennedy, J.G.: "An ultrasonic—EMG transducer for biodynamic research." *J Speech Hear Res, 21*:174-182, 1978.
Wilson, D.K.: *Voice Problems of Children*. Baltimore, Williams and Wilkins, 1972.
Wilson, F.B.: "The voice-disordered child: a descriptive approach." *Lang Speech Hear Services in Schools, 4*: 1972.

Chapter 8

ROUTINE AUDIOMETRIC MEASUREMENT

Michael P. Rosenblatt

THE ROUTINE hearing evaluation should consist of pure tone air conduction and bone conduction testing, speech audiometric testing, and acoustic-impedance measures. This chapter will concentrate on the administration of these tests and interpretation of results. In addition, some attention will be devoted to masking.

PURE TONE AUDIOMETRY

Most basic audiometric measurements are performed by using single-frequency tones called pure tones. The least complex of these measurements are the routine pure tone air conduction and bone conduction tests. Air conduction testing is simply assessment of the auditory system through earphones, while bone conduction testing is inner ear assessment performed with a small bone conduction vibrator, similar to a hearing aid, which is attached to a head band. These tests, when administered properly, will not only detect the presence or absence of a hearing loss, but will furnish the clinician with information regarding the nature of the hearing loss and, in conjunction with case history information, may indicate etiology.

Air Conduction Testing

Before proceeding to the actual mechanics of test administration, it should be pointed out that the experienced clinician does not always strictly adhere to one testing technique. Different patients do not react similarly to all test situations, and the experienced clinician is able to modify his techniques accordingly. The beginner, however, is not yet ready to do so and should follow a strict routine until his skills have been sharpened.

Test Administration

1. Plug in and turn on the audiometer. Allow it to "warm up" for at least ten minutes.

2. Position the patient so that he will be unable to observe the tester. He should not obtain any clues as to presentation of the stimulus.

3. Instruct the patient carefully. It is essential that the task be thoroughly understood. Instructions can be given in the following manner:

"You are going to hear some beeping tones. Some will be high pitched and some will be low pitched (illustrate if necessary). They are going to be fairly loud at first but will eventually become very faint. Whenever you hear a tone, whether it is loud or very faint, please press the button (or raise hand, finger, etc).

Depress the button for as long as you hear the tone, and release it when the tone goes away. Do you hear any better with one ear than the other? We will test that ear first. If both ears are the same you will hear the tones in your right ear first. Are there any questions?"

4. Carefully place the earphones, making sure the diaphragm is directly over the external auditory ear canal. In addition, be sure the earphone marked with red is over the right ear and the blue marked earphone is over the left ear. Some patients have very small or slitlike external auditory canals that will close upon placement of earphones. This may cause test results to show an air/bone gap, when in actuality none exists (air/bone gaps will be discussed later). The clinician should, therefore, inspect the patients ears, and if the canals seal shut when pressure is applied to the pinna, a short length of hollow tubing should be inserted in the canal. Collapsed ear canals occur most often with geriatric patients.

5. It is now time for the actual testing. The procedure involves exploring for and determining threshold. Threshold can be defined as the lowest intensity level at which the stimulus is per-

ceived 50 percent of the time.

6. As mentioned in the instructions, the better ear should be tested first. The reason for this is to save time if masking is needed. Masking will be discussed in a later section. If the patient does not indicate a sensitivity difference between ears, test the right ear first. The rationale behind this is to simply establish a routine, since there is less chance for error in conducting the test and recording the results when the same procedure is followed from test to test.

7. The first frequency to be tested is 1000 Hz because this frequency is near the center of the most sensitive area of the human ear and has been demonstrated to have good test-retest reliability. Following 1000 Hz, test in this order: 2000 Hz, 4000 Hz, 8000 Hz, 1000 Hz, for test-retest reliability, 500 Hz and 250 Hz. Due to the relationship between the wavelength of an 8000 Hz tone and the distance between the earphone diaphragm and eardrum, results at this frequency must be looked at with caution. A hearing loss may be indicated when one does not actually exist. The threshold at 8000 Hz does not really contribute much to the clinical picture, and many audiologists prefer not to test at 8000 Hz.

8. Estimate the patient's threshold and administer the first tonal presentation at a level of 30 dB above the estimated threshold. This will allow the patient to become acquainted with the listening task. For instance, if an individual appears to have normal hearing acuity, begin testing at 30 dB HTL. If a moderate impairment seems present, begin at 70 dB HTL.

9. Present the tone. If the patient does not respond, increase the intensity in 20 dB intervals until a response is obtained. Following the initial response, decrease the intensity by 10 dB and present another tone. If the lower tone is detected, decrease the intensity by another 10 dB. Continue descending until the listener no longer responds. Threshold should be at some level between the last response and the final no response. We have just explored for threshold.

10. Increase the intensity 5 dB from the level where the listener ceased responding. If a response is not obtained, continue as-

cending in 5 dB steps until the tone is again detected. This is the first ascent.

11. Decrease the intensity 10 dB from this most recent response level and present the tone. When the stimulus is no longer audible, ascend in 5 dB steps again.

12. Keep track of the levels at which responses occur. The lowest intensity level at which a response occurs in 2 of 4 ascents is recorded as threshold. Once threshold has been determined, proceed to the next frequency. This procedure is known as the Hughson-Westlake technique (Carhart and Jerger, 1959).

13. When a tone is presented to the ear, it may become inaudible in a very short time. This is known as auditory adaptation. To avoid this phenomenon, each tonal burst should be no more than one or two seconds in duration.

14. The interstimulus interval should be varied from two to five seconds to avoid falling into a rhythmical pattern of presentation. If the clinician does get into a rhythmical pattern, the patient may be able to follow this pattern and respond in anticipation to the tone rather than when he actually hears it.

Bone Conduction

The purpose of bone conduction audiometry is to directly evaluate the function of the cochlea. The outer and middle ears are bypassed when the tone is sent through the bone vibrator. Even if the air conduction pathway is blocked, sound may still be perceived in the cochlea.

There are essentially three modes of bone conduction stimulation, the first being compression bone conduction. Vibrating energy reaching the cochlea causes alternate compressions and expansions of the cochlea shell. These opposite movements force the incompressible cochlea fluid to yield, thus producing a displacement of the basilar membrane (Dirks, 1973). This mode has its greatest effect on the frequencies 1800 Hz and above.

The second mode, referred to as inertia bone conduction, arises from the inertia of the ossicular chain. The inertia of the ossicles during forced vibrations of the skull sets up a relative motion between the stapes and oval window, leading to cochlea stimulation in the same manner as that produced by an air conducted signal (Dirks, 1972). This has its greatest effect on frequencies below 800 Hz.

The third mode deals with the reception of sound energy radiated into the external ear canal. When a vibrating signal is applied to the skull, energy is produced by the walls of the external canal and transmitted to the tympanic membrane (Dirks, 1973). These three modes all contribute to the total bone conduction response.

Testing Procedure

Bone conduction thresholds are determined using the same procedure previously outlined for air conduction. There are, however, some additional factors of which the clinician must be aware when testing bone conduction.

1. When testing bone conduction (without masking), only the better cochlea is being assessed regardless of where the bone vibrator is placed. Therefore, if mastoid placement is used (see 4 below), it is not necessary to test with both the vibrator on the right mastoid process and then on the left mastoid process because the same cochlea will be measured. Also, it is important when giving instructions to tell the patient to respond no matter where the tone is perceived. Some patients feel they should only respond if they hear the tone on the side the vibrator is placed (if mastoid placement is utilized).

2. Do not test bone conduction at 125 Hz and 8000 Hz. The bone vibrator has numerous deficiencies, one of those being a limit in its sound-sending characteristics restricting the number of measureable frequencies. In addition, at 250 Hz, the vibrations are stronger, and the patient may respond to these vibrations without actually hearing the tone. Therefore, bone conduction results at 250 Hz should be viewed with caution, especially if they are inconsistent with other findings.

3. More energy is required to produce sound out of the bone vibrator than the earphones. As a result, the audiometric limits for bone conduction testing are substantially lower than those for air conduction. Bone conduction hearing levels can only be

measured up to 40 or 45 dB HTL at 250 Hz and 65 or 70 dB H TL at the remaining test frequencies. These limits may vary slightly depending upon the audiometer but will not exceed 45 dB H TL at 250 Hz and 70 dB H TL at 500 Hz through 4000 Hz.

4. Bone conduction testing has traditionally been performed with the vibrator placed on the mastoid process of the temporal bone behind the pinna. Placement at the midline of the forehead, however, may be the best site. Three major advantages over mastoid placement have been described. Hart and Naunton (1961) suggested that test-retest reliability is improved with forehead placement. Dirks (1964) and Studebaker (1962) did not, however, find great differences in test-retest reliability between mastoid and forehead placement. There is less intersubject variability, and also, middle ear involvement interfering with bone conduction measurements is decreased with forehead placement. There is an important disadvantage to testing bone conduction thresholds at the midline of the forehead. Approximately 10 dB more intensity is needed to reach threshold here compared with mastoid measurements. This becomes a problem when testing individuals who have a substantial loss of bone conduction sensitivity because, due to the decreased limits for bone conduction testing, the range of measurable hearing is reduced.

5. If mastoid placement is used, the side on which the vibrator is located should not matter since only the better cochlea will be stimulated. For the purpose of establishing a routine, however, place the vibrator behind the ear that exhibits the better air conduction thresholds. This does not necessarily mean that this ear will show better bone conduction thresholds. If the ears are symmetrical, place the vibrator on whichever side you please. When placing the vibrator, be careful to make solid contact with the mastoid bone and avoid touching the pinna. If the bone vibrator is against the pinna, vibrations may arise in the external auditory canal possibly creating an air conduction signal.

6. When testing unmasked bone conduction, do not close off the external auditory canal. Occluding the external canal creates an increase in the loudness of a bone conducted signal in a normal-hearing subject (Dirks, 1973). Bone conduction measures may be

improved by as much as 25–30 dB at 250 Hz and 15 dB at 1000 Hz. Above 1000 Hz, improvement is minimal. This phenomenon is known as the occlusion effect.

Masking

The concept and application of masking is beyond the scope of this text. It is, however, such an integral part of pure tone audiometry that a basic understanding is essential.

When a tone is presented through earphones to one ear at an intensity level greater than 40 dB above the bone conduction threshold of the nontest ear, the tone may cross over the skull and be heard in the opposite ear. The tone will not be perceived in the opposite ear if it is lower than this level because of a reduction in intensity provided by the skull, referred to as interaural attenuation. As opposed to air conduction, interaural attenuation for bone conduction is zero. This means that crossover occurs immediately upon presentation of a bone conducted signal regardless of the intensity level.

The problem crossover presents is obvious. Situations will arise in which the clinician will not know what ear is actually responding to the tone. To resolve this dilemma, he must use masking. Masking is simply the presentation of noise into the nontest ear to eliminate it from participating. The preferred noise for masking pure tones is narrow-band noise. This type of noise is most effective because the majority of its energy is concentrated around the frequency of the test tone.

When to Mask

Since interaural attenuation for air conduction is approximately 40 dB, masking is not necessary until this level is exceeded. The rule for air conduction testing is to mask the nontest ear whenever the signal presented to the test ear exceeds the bone conduction threshold in the nontest ear by more than 40 dB (Sanders, 1972). Although interaural attenuation for bone conduction is zero, it is not necessary to always mask when testing bone conduction. Appropriate diagnostic information can be obtained if the nontest ear is masked whenever the air conduction threshold of the test ear exceeds the bone conduction threshold by more than 10 dB.

How to Mask

There are a number of different formulas and procedures that deal with the appropriate amount of masking and its administration. The procedure advocated here is one proposed by Hood (1960). The noise is introduced into the nontest ear at an effective level of 10 dB above the threshold of the nontest ear. Effective level can be regarded as the threshold shift in dB produced in the masked ear by a given amount of noise (Sanders, 1972). The dial readings of many audiometers are calibrated in effective masking for narrow band noise. If this is not the case, effective levels can be determined through computation. The noise level is increased in 10 dB steps each time the patient responds to the tone. If the patient does not respond to the tone, the tone intensity is raised in 5 dB steps without any further increase in the noise level until a response is again obtained. This procedure is continued until three or four successive responses are obtained at one threshold level. This is a fairly simple and widely used technique.

In speech audiometry, masking is unnecessary unless the speech signal is presented to the test ear at a level greater than 50 dB above the average of the pure tone bone conduction thresholds at 500 Hz, 1000 Hz, and 2000 Hz of the nontest ear. The procedure simply involves placing a sufficient amount of noise (effective) in the nontest ear to assure that it is not participating. The preferred masking noises for speech audiometry are white noise and speech noise.

The Audiogram

Results from air conduction and bone conduction testing are recorded on a graph called an audiogram. The clinician records these results separately for each ear with various standardized symbols. Right ear results should be recorded in red, and blue should be used for the left ear.

Figure 8-1 shows a typical audiogram form and the appropriate symbols. The frequencies are along the abscissa and intensity levels are along the ordinate. If a patient's air conduction threshold at 1000 Hz for the right ear is 20 dB, the clinician simply plots a red circle at the point on the audiogram where 20 dB intersects 1000 Hz. Results for all test frequencies are recorded in a similar manner using the correct symbols. Bone conduction results should be plotted slightly to the side of the point where frequency intersects intensity. There is also an area on the audiogram form designated for speech audiometric results.

Audiogram Interpretation

The audiogram provides information pertaining to how well or poorly an individual hears and the nature of hearing impair-

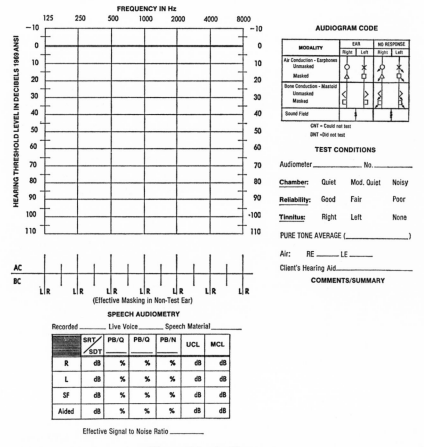

Figure 8-1. Audiogram.

ment. Hearing losses range anywhere from slight to profound. A suggested guideline for interpreting degree of hearing loss is as follows: −10 to 14 dB normal, 15 to 25 dB slight, 26 to 40 dB mild, 41 to 55 dB moderate, 56 to 70 dB marked, 71 to 90 dB severe, above 90 dB profound. There are three types of hearing losses: conductive, sensorineural, and mixed.

The conductive hearing loss results from pathology or malfunctioning of the outer and/or middle ear with a normal inner ear (Newby, 1958). Since bone conduction measures essentially only inner ear sensitivity while air conduction assesses the entire auditory system, an individual with a conductive hearing loss will show normal bone conduction thresholds but exhibit a loss by air conduction.

When the separation between the bone conduction and air conduction thresholds for the same ear, commonly referred to as the air/bone gap, exceeds 10 dB a conductive component is said to exist. Generally, the conductive hearing loss is characterized by an equal amount of air conduction loss at all frequencies, with

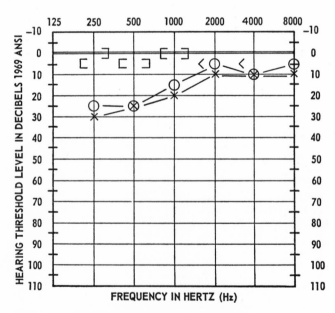

Figure 8-2. Bilateral otitis media.

a slightly greater loss possibly present at the lower frequencies. In most cases, the conditions that cause conductive hearing losses are accessible to medical or surgical treatment. Figures 8-2 and 8-3 illustrate two types of conductive hearing losses.

The sensorineural hearing loss is essentially due to pathology of the inner ear. The audiogram will show a loss of hearing sensitivity by both air and bone conduction with air/bone gaps being no greater than 10 dB. In other words, there is approximately an equal loss in both bone and air conduction sensitivity. This type of hearing loss is usually, but not always, characterized by a greater sensitivity loss in the higher frequencies than in the lower frequencies. Figures 8-4, 8-5, and 8-6 illustrate three sensorineural hearing losses.

The mixed impairment involves both middle (and/or outer) and inner ear pathology. The audiogram is characterized by some loss by bone conduction with air/bone gaps exceeding 10 dB. A mixed impairment may also exhibit an audiogram with a conductive loss in the lower frequencies and a sensorineural loss in the higher frequencies. Figure 8-7 represents a mixed hearing loss.

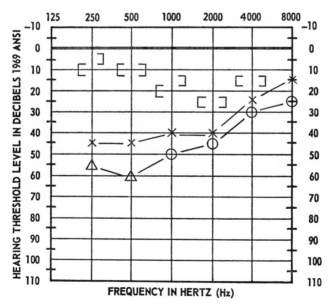

Figure 8-3.   Bilateral otosclerosis.

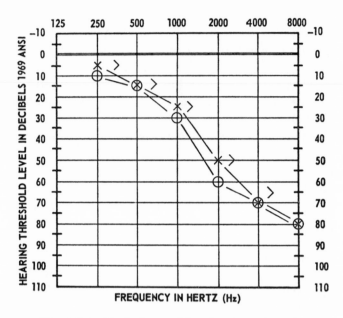

Figure 8-4. Typical type of loss due to presbycusis.

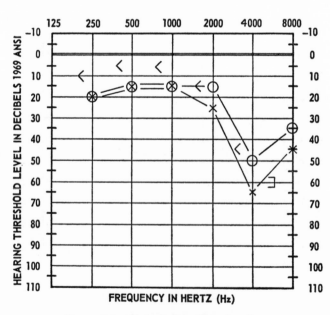

Figure 8-5. Noise induced hearing loss.

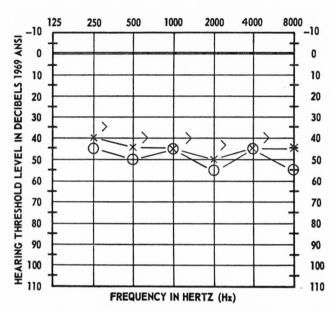

Figure 8-6. Flat sensorineural hearing loss.

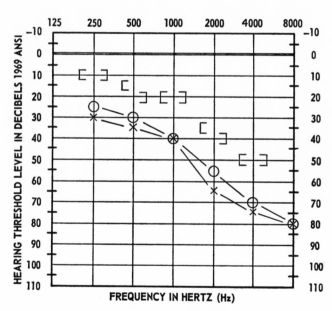

Figure 8-7. Mixed hearing loss.

The illustrations provided in this section are intended to give the reader a general idea of the audiological picture that a certain pathology may present. It must be noted, however, that pathology from patient to patient does not always present the typical picture. Results, in fact, may be quite variable.

SPEECH AUDIOMETRY

Speech audiometric measures supplement pure tone findings and provide additional diagnostic, rehabilitative, and prognostic information. There are two basic aspects of speech audiometry. They are speech reception threshold testing and measurement of speech discrimination.

Speech Reception Threshold

The speech reception threshold is a measure of the lowest intensity level at which an individual can barely identify simple speech materials (Berger, 1971). A great deal of research has gone into the development of materials for both speech reception and speech discrimination testing. The major criteria for the development of speech reception tests were familiarity of words, phonetic dissimilarity, normal sampling of English sounds, and homogeneity with respect to audibility (Hudgins et al., 1947).

The tests most commonly used today are the "CID" — W1 and W2 spondaic word lists. They use lists of two-syllable words with equal stress on each syllable known as spondee words. An example of such a word is *airplane*. These tests can be administered on tape or by live voice.

Test Administration

There are a number of different procedures for determining the speech reception threshold. The procedure advocated is very similar to that for obtaining pure tone thresholds. The step by step procedure follows.

1. Inform the patient that he will be hearing some two-syllable words which start out fairly loud but will gradually decrease in loudness. The patient is to repeat what he hears, guessing if necessary.

2. Test the better ear first. Begin presenting spondees (two-

syllable words with equal stress on each syllable) at a level 30 dB above the average of the pure tone thresholds at 500, 1000, and 2000 Hz. This is referred to as the pure tone average. When presenting the spondees, be sure the VU meter on the audiometer peaks at zero for the first syllable. If the test is administered by live voice, the clinician should be no further than 10 inches from the audiometer microphone.

3. Present two spondees at this initial level and descend in 10 dB steps, presenting two words at each level. Continue this process until the patient does not repeat any words correctly.

4. Increase the intensity in 5 dB steps until the patient is able to repeat two of four spondees.

5. Decrease the intensity in 10 dB steps until the patient can no longer repeat two of four spondees.

6. Repeat step 4.

7. The lowest intensity level where the patient is able to repeat two of four spondees (50%) is the speech reception threshold (SRT).

Clinical Application

The value of the speech reception threshold lies mainly in confirming pure tone findings and predicting hearing handicap. The speech reception threshold should correspond very closely to the average of the pure tone thresholds at 500 Hz, 1000 Hz, and 2000 Hz (Pure Tone Average). If the patient exhibits a steeply sloping pure tone audiogram, a two-frequency pure tone average may be used. The difference between these measures should be no greater than 10 dB. If there is a large discrepancy, it may suggest either an error in test administration by the clinician (pure tone or speech), a failure of the patient to adequately perform the task, or a simulated hearing loss.

The speech reception threshold also serves as a guideline for describing degree of hearing handicap. Persons exhibiting slight and mild hearing losses for speech should only have difficulty hearing soft speech. Individuals with moderate losses will experience difficulty hearing normal conversational speech while those with marked impairments have frequent difficulty with loud speech.

The severely impaired patient may hear only shouted or

amplified speech, and those with profound losses have difficulty with even amplified speech.

Speech Discrimination Testing Materials

There have been a substantial number of materials developed for testing speech discrimination. The original criteria for development were that the words should be familiar, monosyllabic, and phonetically balanced. From these criteria the Harvard Psycho Acoustic Laboratory PB 50 lists (Egan, 1948) and the Central Institute for the Deaf Auditory Test W22 (Hirsh et al., 1952) developed. Next to develop were monosyllables of the consonant-vowel-consonant type, which arose from the concept that it was possible to develop lists of words that were only in certain respects phonemically balanced (Lehiste and Peterson, 1959). The most prominent of these lists is the Northwestern University Auditory Test No. 6. All these tests are referred to as "open response sets" in that they require the patient to repeat what he hears without being allowed to choose among a number of items. Not all test materials are of the "open response set" type. The Fairbanks Rhyme (Fairbanks, 1958) and Modified Rhyme Tests are two multiple choice tests: The former consists of 50 sets of five rhyming monosyllables, and the later consists of twenty-five monosyllables differing only in the initial consonant and twenty-five monosyllables differing only in the initial consonant and twenty-five differing in the final consonant. Another nonopen response set test is one composed of words grouped together without regard for syntax or meaning known as the Synthetic Sentence Identification Test (SSI) (Speaks and Jerger, 1965). These three tests are "closed response sets" because the patient is allowed to select the correct response from a given number of items.

There is presently no one test that has gained universal acceptance among audiologists. The monosyllabic word lists described in the initial paragraph of this section have, however, received a more widespread application (Tillman and Olsen, 1973).

Test Administration

The word discrimination tests should be administered at a level where the patient is most likely to attain his maximum score.

This level is usually between 30 dB to 50 dB above the speech reception threshold of the test ear. The tests are, therefore, most often given at a level of 40 dB above the speech reception threshold. If this level is uncomfortably loud it is acceptable to administer the test at the patient's most comfortable level.

It is essential that before presenting each actual item a carrier phrase such as "Say the Word" be given to alert the patient to the test. The final word of this carrier phrase should be peaked at zero on the audiometer's VU meter. The patient may be allowed to respond by simply repeating what he hears or recording responses on paper. The number correct is totaled and this score is converted into a percentage.

Clinical Application

Speech discrimination measures serve as an aid in site of lesion diagnosis, determining hearing aid candidacy, and in describing hearing handicap. Goetzinger (1972) suggests the following guideline for interpreting the results:

1. 90–100%—Excellent, normal limits.
2. 75–90%—Slight difficulty in speech understanding, comparable to listening over a telephone.
3. 60–75%—Moderate difficulty in speech understanding.
4. 50–60%—Poor discrimination, marked difficulty in following conversation.
5. Below 50%—Very poor discrimination, probably unable to follow running speech.

Speech discrimination ability manifests itself differently with regard to pathology. Word discrimination ability in patients with conductive impairments is usually 90 percent or better (Goetzinger, 1972). If a patient has a conductive hearing loss and poor speech discrimination, the clinician should suspect a concurrent pathology of the hearing mechanism or a possible error in pure tone test results. Individuals with presbycusis (hearing impairment due to advanced age) may show severely reduced discrimination scores, which are not commensurate with pure tone thresholds. Patients with eighth nerve tumors may also show this phenomenon. Another important characteristic of individuals with eighth nerve tumors is that, when the intensity of the speech signal is gradually increased beyond the level of maximum performance, there may be a drastic decrease in the word discrimination score. This has proven to be an extremely valuable diagnostic tool. In addition, various distorted and difficult speech tasks are being used for the evaluation of central nervous system function. A discussion of these, however, is beyond the scope of this text.

The final area of clinical application lies within hearing aid candidacy and hearing aid evaluation. Speech discrimination measures have long been used in hearing aid evaluations as the primary source for differentiating between hearing aids. Speech discrimination measures alert the clinician as to how much benefit a person may obtain from a hearing aid. An individual with good speech discrimination is most likely a good hearing aid candidate, while an individual with very low discrimination scores is probably a poor candidate. The audiologist should not, however, make a decision for the recommendation of a hearing aid based solely on low discrimination scores. Individuals with reduced discrimination scores often synthesize sentence material quite well with amplification and, hence, receive a good deal of benefit from a hearing aid (Goetzinger, 1972).

ACOUSTIC IMPEDANCE

During the past decade, acoustic impedance measurements have changed the practice of clinical audiology. Acoustic impedance refers specifically to the resistance to movement of the tympanic membrane when stimulated by sound pressure (Northern, 1971).

Acoustic impedance measures supply a direct, objective measure of middle ear function. There are three separate types of measures included in acoustic impedance testing. These measures are tympanometry, static compliance, and stapedius reflex thresholds. Before proceeding to a discussion of these measures, a brief description of instrumentation is necessary.

Instrumentation

The modern acoustic impedance bridge consists of a headset and a variety of dials, meters, and controls. The headset includes a head band with a single earphone plugged into a standard audio-meter output jack and a metal transducer box with three tubes connected to a probe tip. The three tubes connect to three holes in the probe tip through which are presented a probe tone, vari-able air pressure system, and a pickup microphone system, which measures reflected probe tone signal intensity (Northern, 1975).

The manometer (air pressure meter) indicates the existing air pressure in the outer ear canal between the probe tip and the tympanic membrane. The air pressure knob is used for increasing and decreasing this pressure. The long scale on the bridge is the compliance or cursor scale, which allows readings of absolute values of compliance. The balance meter indicates relative changes in compliance. Adjustment of the compliance knob changes the intensity of the probe tone signal. Lastly, the sensi-tivity knob influences the sensitivity of the pickup microphone system.

Tympanometry

Tympanometry is a technique for determining how the com-pliance of the middle ear system changes in response to variation in the air pressure at the lateral surface of the tympanic mem-brane (Jerger, 1975). A graph called a tympanogram is plotted from this measure. The shape of the tympanogram supplies valu-able diagnostic information regarding middle ear status. Figures 8-8 through 8-12 illustrate the basic types of tympanograms and pathologies they indicate.

Static Compliance

Static compliance measurements compare differences in equivalent volume between the most compliant ear drum position and most taut position. A measure of ≥ 1.6 cc indicates excessive ear drum mobility, .26cc to 1.5cc is normal and a measure $\leq .25$cc indicates stiffness.

Stapedius Reflex

The stapedius muscle of the middle ear contracts reflexively in response to intense sound. The reflex is a bilateral phenome-non, meaning that sound in either ear causes both muscles to con-

TYMPANOGRAM

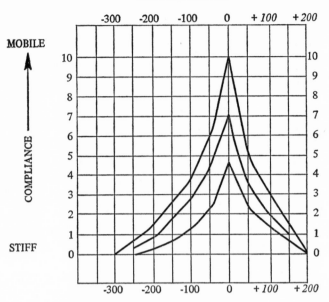

Figure 8-8. Normal tympanogram.

TYMPANOGRAM

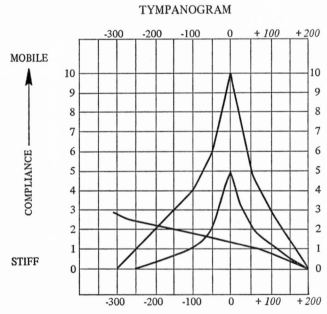

Figure 8-9. Tympanogram indicative of otitis media or impacted cerumen.

TYMPANOGRAM

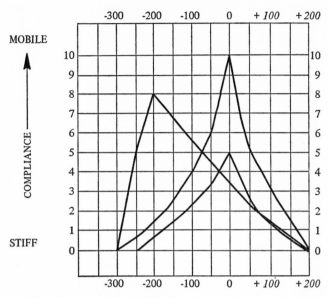

Figure 8-10. Tympanogram indicative of excessive negative pressure.

TYMPANOGRAM

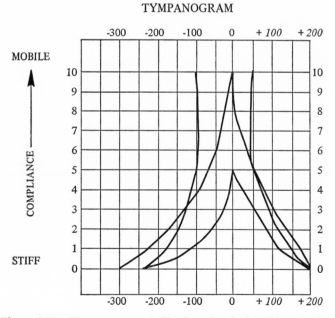

Figure 8-11. Tympanogram indicative of ossicular discontinuity.

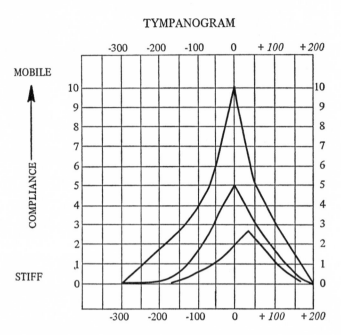

Figure 8-12. Tympanogram indicative of otosclerosis.

tract. The intensity levels at which contraction occurs can aid in differential diagnosis. The average level above the pure tone threshold (sensation level) that the reflex occurs is 85 dB with the normal range being approximately 60–100 dB (Jerger, 1975). Individuals with cochlea hearing impairments should exhibit the reflex at reduced sensation levels, i.e. less than 60 dB above the pure tone threshold. In patients with conductive hearing losses or eighth nerve lesions, the reflex should be absent (no response at upper limits of the audiometer) or present at a normal sensation level (within 60–100 dB SL) but elevated reflex threshold level. The reflex is at an elevated level if the threshold is above 100 dB. In other words, if the reflex threshold is at 110 dB and the pure tone threshold is 25 dB, the reflex is occurring at a normal sensation level (85 dB) but at an elevated reflex threshold level. Reflex abnormalities of this type, may, however, sometimes be seen in normals.

Impedance Administration

The following is a description of procedures for test administration on one type of impedance bridge.

Tympanometry

1. Place probe tip in ear obtaining hermetic seal.
2. Adjust pressure to +200 (Sensitivity should be no 1 or T).
3. Record the CC value from the complicance scale (C_1). it is on far right hand reading.
4. Reduce pressure. Note compliance change at +200, +100, 0, maximum change, −100, and −200.

Static Compliance

1. Adjust pressure to +200.
2. Using the compliance knob adjust the balance meter needle until it is at black 0 (middle).
3. Record the CC value from the compliance scale (C_1).
4. Reduce pressure to the point of maximum compliance.
5. Using the compliance knob, adjust the balance meter needle until it is at the black zero again.
6. Record the CC value from the compliance scale (C_2).
7. Compute $C_2 - C^1 =$ Static compliance.

Acoustic (Stapedius) Reflex

1. Set pressure at point of maximum compliance.
2. Change sensitivity to R or 3.
3. Using compliance knob, adjust balance meter needle until it is at or near black 0 (middle).
4. Present tone signal.
5. Watch balance meter for deflection of approximately one hash mark.
6. Record lowest intensity level at which deflection occurs.

References

Berger, K.: Speech Audiometry. In D. Rose (Ed.): *Audiological Assessment*. Englewood Cliffs, N.J.: Prentice-Hall, Inc., 1971.

Carhart, R. and Jerger, J.: Preferred Method for Clinical Determination of Pure Tone Thresholds. *J Speech Hearing Dis, 24,* 330-345, 1959.

Davis, H.: Audiometry: Pure Tone and Simple Speech Tests. In H. Davis and S.R. Silverman (Eds.): *Hearing and Deafness*. New York:

Holt, Rinehart and Winston, Inc., 1947.

Davis, H.: Hearing Handicap, Standards for Hearing, and Medicolegal Rules. In H. Davis and S.R. Silverman (Eds.): *Hearing and Deafness.* New York: Holt, Rinehart and Winston, Inc., 1947.

Dirks, D.D.: Bone Conduction Measurements. In J. Jerger (Ed.): *Modern Developments in Audiology.* New York: Academic Press, 1973.

Dirks, D.D.: Clinical Measurement of Bone Conduction. In J. Katz (Ed.): *Handbook of Clinical Audiology.* Baltimore: Williams and Wilkins Co., 1972.

Dirks, D.D. and Malmquist, C.: Comparison of Frontal and Mastoid Bone Conduction Thresholds in Various Conduction Lesions. *J Speech Hearing Res, 12,* 725-746, 1969.

Dirks, D.D.: Factors Related to Bone Conduction Reliability. *Arch Otolaryngol, 79,* 551-558, 1964.

Egan, J.P.: Articulation Testing Methods, *Laryngoscope, 58,* 955-991, 1948.

Fairbanks, G.: Test of Phonemic Differentiation: The Rhyme Test. *J Acoust Soc Amer. 30,* 596-600, 1958.

Feldman, A.: Acoustic Impedance-Admittance Measurements. In L. Bradford (Ed.): *Physiological Measures of Audio-Vestibular System.* New York: Academic Press, 1975.

Goetzinger, C.: Word Discrimination Testing. In J. Katz (Ed.): *Handbok of Clinical Audiology.* Baltimore: Williams and Wilkins Co., 1972.

Hart, C. and Naunton, R.F.: Frontal Bone Conduction Tests in Clinical Audiometry. *Laryngoscope, 71,* 24-29, 1961.

Hirsh, I.J., Davis, H., Silverman, S.R., Reynolds, E.G., Eldert, E., and Bensen, R.W.: Development of Materials for Speech Audiometry. *J Speech Hearing Dis, 17,* 321-337, 1952.

Hood, J.D.: The Principles and Practice of Bone Conduction Audiometry. *Laryngoscope, 70,* 1211-1228, 1960.

Hopkinson, N.: Speech Reception Threshold. In J. Katz (Ed.): *Handbook of Clinical Audiology.* Baltimore: Williams and Wilkins Co., 1972.

House, A., Williams, C., Hecker, M., and Kryter, K.: Articulation Testing Methods: Consonantal Differentiation with a Closed-Response Set. *J Acoust Soc Amer, 37,* 158-166, 1965.

Hudgins, C.V., Hawkins, J.E., Jr. Karlin, J.E. and Stevens, S.S.: The Development of Recorded Auditory Tests for Measuring Hearing Loss for Speech. *Laryngoscope, 57,* 57-89, 1947.

Jerger, J.: Diagnostic Use of Impedance Measures. In J. Jerger (Ed.): *Handbook of Clinical Impedance Audiometry.* New York: American Electromedics Corporation, 1975.

Jerger, J.: Foreword. In J. Jerger (Ed.): *Handbook of Clinical Imped-*

ance Audiometry. New York: American Electromedics Corporation, 1975.

Lehiste, I. and Peterson, G.E.: Linguistic Considerations in the study of Speech Intelligibility. *J Acoust Soc Amer, 31,* 280-286 (1959).

Newby, H.A.: *Audiology.* New York: Appleton-Century-Crofts, 1958.

Northern, J.: Clinical Application of Acoustic Impedance Measurements. In W. Hemenway and L. Bergston (Eds.): *The Otolaryngologic Clinics of North America.* Philadelphia: W.B. Saunders Co., 1971.

Northern, J.: Clinical Measurement Procedures. In J. Jerger (Ed.): *Handbook of Clinical Impedance Audiometry.* New York: American Electromedics Corporation, 1975.

Price, L.L.: Pure-Tone Audiometry. In D. Rose (Ed.): *Audiological Assessment.* Englewood Cliffs, N.J.: Prentice-Hall, Inc., 1971.

Sanders, J.: Masking. In J. Katz (Ed.): *Handbook of Clinical Audiology.* Baltimore: Williams and Wilkins Co., 1972.

Speaks, C. and Jerger, J.: Method for Measurement of Speech Identification. *J Speech Hearing Res, 8,* 185-194, 1965.

Studebaker, G.A.: Auditory Masking. In J. Jerger (Ed.): *Modern Developments in Audiology.* New York: Academic Press, 1973.

Studebaker, G.A.: Placement of Vibrator in Bone Conduction Testing. *J Speech Hearing Res, 5,* 321-331, 1962.

Tillman, T. and Olsen, M.: Speech Audiometry, In J. Jerger (Ed.): *Modern Developments in Audiology,* New York: Academic Press, 1973.

Tonndorf, J.: Bone Conduction: Studies in Experimental Animals. *Acta Otolaryngol Suppl, 213,* 1966.

Chapter 9

INFANT HEARING TESTING

Linda I. Seestedt

INTRODUCTION

Early identification and remedial intervention of a hearing impaired child can maximize his opportunity to develop adequate speech and language. A child with a hearing problem must be identified before the "critical period" for language acquisition has passed. Most children acquire grammatical speech and possess a basis for the development of adult grammar within a period of twenty-four months, beginning before one and one-half years and completed by three and one-half years of age (Marge, 1972). During this time, both hearing and the age of the child play key roles in language learning. A hearing impaired child must have the same opportunity to develop speech and language as a normal child. Auditory development must occur as near as possible to its appropriate chronological sequence. Failure to identify a hearing impaired child during his first year of life will cause retardation not only in language acquisition but also in educational and sociological development.

The audiologic assessment of an infant is a necessary procedure to ensure the effective use of amplification. Further, the success of a rehabilitation program is dependent on the early detection of a child's hearing problem and good audiologic intervention.

An attempt is made in this chapter to provide information regarding the auditory development of the infant and to discuss various procedures that may be used to assess his hearing sensitivity.

The effective evaluation of an infant's hearing takes both skill

278

and experience. It is hoped that the information provided in this chapter can assist the beginning clinician in obtaining the background necessary to complement his clinical training.

AUDITORY DEVELOPMENT

To accurately assess the hearing of infants and young children, one must have a firm, clear understanding of the development of an auditory function. It is critical that a clinician know expected auditory behavior from an infant at a particular age level. Literature dealing with the physiological development of the human hearing mechanism is extensive. Information directly concerned with auditory behavior in infants, however, is sparse. A brief discussion of auditory development in man at prenatal, neonatal, and infant stages will be presented for review.

Prenatal

Evidence that man is able to "hear" *in utero* and react to that stimulation provides the first stage in the developmental schema. Research in the area of prenatal response to sound is a natural starting point for work with newborns and older groups of infants.

Vasiliu (1968) pointed out that a child is ready to hear in the fifth month of gestation when both the cochlea and sense end organ have structurally reached full adult size (Elliot and Elliot, 1964; Eisenberg, 1969). Investigations done on human fetuses provided evidence of this (Johansson et al., 1964; and Dwornicka et al., 1964).

Studies with premature infants also point out that neurologically the auditory system is intact and operating at birth. Premature newborns respond both automatically and behaviorally to different stimuli (Eisenberg et al., 1970, 1964).

Neonatal (0–1 Month)

Since it is well documented that an infant is capable of hearing at birth, much of the present research centers on parameters of stimuli and their differential effect on the response pattern. It is clear that identification of a hearing problem, whatever a subject's age, depends on the kinds of signals used and the ways in which they are employed (Eisenberg, 1971). Intensity, frequency, and duration needed to elicit responses from neonates have been explored by numerous investigations. By observing newborn responses to different stimuli, a broader understanding of auditory behavior, its development, and refinement can be obtained.

Intensity

The parameter of intensity plays a distinctive role in eliciting neonatal behavioral response to sound. Response patterns are known to vary in contrast to high or low intensity sounds. Investigations as early as 1882 examined and sought to explain responses of newborns to strong auditory stimulation. Later studies substantiated the need for intense stimuli to elicit detectable behavioral responses in newborns (Eisenberg, 1965; Ling et al., 1970; Downs and Sterritt, 1967).

Frequency

The parameter of frequency also exerts differential effects on the incidence of neonatal response to auditory stimuli. Eisenberg et al. (1964) indicated that "frequency is undoubtedly one determinant of response pattern." In reviewing the literature, types of stimuli employed have ranged from clackers (Hardy et al., 1959) to pop guns (Froding, 1966).

Data obtained by various investigators using pure tones have become rather speculative. It has been found that a pure tone is not an effective stimulus for use with newborns (Ling, et al., 1970; Heron and Jacobs, 1968; Taylor and Mencher, 1972). It is generally considered that a broad band stimulus is the most effective for eliciting observable auditory behavior from newborn infants. Certain mixtures of tones, however, also elicit unique behavior not observed with other stimuli. This phenomena has been labeled a range-dependent mechanism for acoustic processing. Low frequencies and high frequencies have different functional properties. Eisenberg et al. (1970) pointed out that these range-dependent differences in infants are reflected in the kinds of sounds we find annoying. Police sirens, alarm signals, etc. are stimuli that have unpleasant connotations; likewise, they are high frequency sounds. A tendency to respond to high frequency signals both in infancy and later in life may be due to pre-adapted inborn systems.

Conversely, it has been found (Birns et al., 1965) that in newborns a low frequency tone (150 Hz) is an effective soothing signal. Turkewitz et al. (1972) found that a mixture of low tones (250–500 Hz) was the only stimulus to significantly affect the heart rate. Eisenberg (1969) further pointed out that low frequencies are inhibitors of distress and generally evoked gross motor activity.

Duration

Duration of a signal plays an important role in eliciting a positive behavioral response. It has been found that the number of responses per infant increase with bursts of longer duration. (Eisenberg, 1965; Ling, 1972) .

Infant (1–12 Months)

As an infant matures, his responses to auditory stimuli become more reliable, thus making the presence of a possible hearing impairment more readily identifiable. Unfortunately, literature dealing with auditory development in infants is limited. Available research points out that at four weeks of age an infant is startled by sound (Griffiths, 1954). A moro reflex is present at this age; however, an eyeblink and opening of the eyes are dominant behavior (Waldon, 1973). At eight weeks of age an infant is no longer disturbed by loud sounds (Gesell and Amatruda, 1947). Presumably, he begins to learn what is important in his environment (Hardy, 1965). Murphy (1969) contends that as early as the third week after birth an infant ceases to respond to sounds consistently present in his environment, but will startle to uncommon noise. By eight to twelve weeks a child begins to attune to the human voice. He has begun to discriminate and direct his attention. A three-month-old child may begin to search for sound by using his eyes (Griffiths, 1954) . At four months head movements are apparent as the infant explores his auditory world. Further, he responds to stimuli with varying facial expressions

(Frisina, 1973). At five months an infant rolls his eyes and moves his head toward the sound source (Waldon, 1973). At twenty-four weeks a head-turning response is very marked in infants; by seven months Waldon (1974) points out that this response occurs in 100 percent of the cases. From the age of eight to twelve months head turning is the primary response. In many children localization is done with smiling and expressions of comfort (Waldon, 1973).

THE CASE HISTORY

Prior to the actual hearing testing of an infant, a case history interview should be obtained. Parental observation, prenatal, birth, medical and developmental history, as well as speech and language must be recorded. The need for a good case history report is supported by the fact that current behavioral methods for testing infants provide sketchy clinical information. Further, results obtained are dependent upon infant cooperation. Knowledge of a child's background may support the diagnosis of a hearing problem. Various illnesses and trauma to which a child is exposed *in utero* as well as postnatally may cause hearing impairment. A high risk register for hearing loss has been established by the Joint Committee for Infant Hearing Screening.

The criteria for High Risk for Hearing Impairment are the presence of one or more of the following:

A. History of hereditary childhood hearing impairment
B. Rubella or other nonbacterial intrauterine fetal infection
C. Defects of the ear, nose, and throat
D. Birthweight less than 1500 grams
E. Bilirubin level greater than 20 mb/100 ml serum.

These criteria have been found to be effective in identifying 60 to 70 percent of those children born deaf (Mencher, 1976).

INFANT TESTING PROCEDURES

Procedures to assess the hearing sensitivity of older children and adults are well documented and provide conclusive information. Conversely, standard audiometric techniques cannot be used with the infant because of his immature development.

The pediatric hearing assessment is an ongoing process. Conclusive audiologic information can rarely be obtained on an infant in one test session. This necessitates the clinician's use of a battery of procedures. Behavioral as well as electrophysiologic techniques, having proven clinical utility for infants zero to one year of age, are discussed below.

Behavior Observation Audiology

As an alternative to conventional adult procedures, infants are usually tested with an observational technique. With the presentation of a stimulus, a change in the infant's ongoing behavior is noted and credited as a response. This form of testing, called behavior observation audiometry (BOA), is the most widely practiced clinical procedure used with infants today.

A number of variables must be controlled in order for BOA to be an efficient method. As with any hearing testing procedure, equipment must be calibrated. Further, the stimuli employed must be appropriate and effective in eliciting infant behavior. Several investigators (Mendel, 1968; Hoversten and Moncur, 1969; Thompson and Thompson, 1972; Waldon, 1973; Thompson and Weber, 1974; Seestedt and Bess, 1974) have shown that broad band noise, narrow band noise, and speech stimuli are more effective than pure tones in eliciting auditory responses from infants zero to twelve months. Also, because of the nature of the test procedure, threshold values obtained are well above adult levels and influenced by the chronological age of the child. Moderately intense signals must be presented to elicit reflexive responses.

A localization response can be observed in a normal child between the ages of four and six months. As stated earlier, a head turn in response to a sound is a very marked behavior by age six months. It is at this age level that more specific information can be obtained regarding a child's auditory functioning. Less intense stimuli are needed in order to elicit auditory behavior. Further, visual reinforcement can be used to increase and maintain responsiveness. Using localization as a criterion for an auditory response and reinforcing that localization with a visual stimuli are the basis for conditioned orientating reflex (COR) (Suzuki and Ogiba, 1961). In this procedure a child is seated between two loud speakers each having connected visual stimuli.

It has been found that COR increases auditory localization in infants, therefore making the assessment of hearing more dependable and satisfactory.

Liden and Kankkunen (1969) reported a variation of the COR test called visual reinforcement audiometry (VRA). In this procedure a child is reinforced visually for any alerting response such as investigatory behavior, localization, reflexes such as APR and spontaneous responses such as vocalizations or smiles. Matkin and Thomas (1975) found that VRA can rule out all but a minimal loss of hearing in the better ear in children nine to twelve months of age.

Behavior observational procedures give us more reliable information with the increasing age of the infant. However, the limitations of this technique are evident. As with most soundfield methods, the hearing of the better ear is assessed. It is difficult to substantiate a unilateral loss through this procedure. Further, depending on the stimulus used, there is danger of missing high frequency impairments and underestimating the degree of hearing loss.

Electrophysiologic Measurements

Electroacoustic Impedance is a necessary part of any pediatric hearing assessment. This objective measurement provides information about the status of the conductive mechanism and corroborative evidence about auditory sensitivity and sensorineural levels (Hodgson, 1978). A complete description of this procedure is explained in the preceding chapter. Research done with infants in the area of impedance testing reveals tympanometry to be a dependable measurement (Keith, 1973). Several investigators (Keith, 1975; Cannon, et al. 1974; Robertson, et al. 1968), however, report that the acoustic stapedial reflex is not a dependable measure in infants zero to twelve months of age when used alone.

Impedance has its limitations, the primary one being that an infant must remain quiet and relatively immobile during the test period. A skilled clinician experienced in child testing should be available for this procedure. Lastly, it should be pointed out that tympanometry and acoustic stapedial reflex measurements must be complemented by a behavioral test battery; only then can results be interpreted and diagnosis made.

Electrocochleography (ECoG)

A second electrophysiologic test that is gaining recognition for use with infants is electrocochleography. Electrocochleography is a direct measure of the peripheral system. An electrode is placed in the external canal wall or trans-tympanically on the cochlear promontory. A ground and indifferent electrode are placed on the forehead and mastoid, respectively. Sound is delivered via a horn. Filtered (third octave) clicks at a rate of 10 per second at the octave frequencies 500–8000 Hz are utilized. The electrodes record cochleographic potentials generated within the cochlea or VIII nerve. The action potential, which is generated by the volley firings of the fibers in the auditory nerve (Dallos, 1973), is the most widely used electrical potential clinically. An electrophysiologic audiogram analogous to the standard behavioral audiogram can be obtained with good agreement (Eggermont et al., 1974; Naughton and Zerlin, 1976).

The advantages of ECoG are evident; it is an objective tool that can reliably measure the hearing sensitivity of an infant. The major disadvantage of this procedure is that general anesthesia is necessary when infants are tested, requiring medical intervention.

Brainstem Evoked Response (BSER)

Brainstem evoked response is an objective hearing test procedure that records neural activity of the auditory nerve and brainstem nuclei.

A target electrode is placed on the vertex with a ground at the forehead and a companion at the earlobe. The stimulus used is a click or extremely brief tone presented two and one-half to ten times per second. All procedures are identical to electrocochleography except for the placement of the target electrode. In interpreting results, the potentials recorded are averaged, and the peaks generated refer to different areas from the VIII nerve to the medial geniculate and primary auditory cortex. Examination of the fifth wave or peak, speculated to arise from the inferior colliculus, is most useful for audiologic purposes. The child being tested can either be awake or asleep; no sedation is necessary in this procedure. BSER is a useful audiologic measurement.

Summary

The beginning clinician should have a thorough knowledge of infant testing procedures, a firm basis in auditory, speech, and language development and as much exposure to actual infant testing as possible. With this background, a student should develop into a capable clinician confident in his ability to assess the hearing of infants.

References

Birns, B., Blank, M., Bridger, W., and Escalona, C.: Behavioral inhibition in neonates produced by auditory stimuli. *Child Dev, 36*:639-644, 1965.

Cannon, S., Smith, K., and Reece, C., et al.: Middle ear measurements in neonates: A normative study. Presentation, American Speech & Hearing Association, 1974.

Dallos, P.: *The Auditory Periphery.* New York, Academic Press, 1973.

Downs, M. and Sterritt, G.: A guide to newborn and infant hearing screening programs. *Arch Otolaryngol, 85*:37-44, 1967.

Dwornicka, B., Jasienska, A., Smolarz, W., and Wawryk, R.: Attempt of determining the fetal reactions to acoustic stimulation. *Acta Otolaryngol, 57*:571-574, 1964.

Eggermont, J., Odenthal, D., Schmidt, P., et al.: Electrocochleography. Basic principles and clinical applications. *Acta Otolaryngol,* suppl 316, Leiden 1974.

Eisenberg, R., Griffin, E., Coursin, D., and Hunter, M.: Auditory, behavior in the human neonate: A preliminary report. *J Speech Hear Res, 7:* 245-269, 1964.

Eisenberg, R.: Auditory behavior in the human neonate: 1. Methodologic problems and the logical design of research procedures. *Journal of Auditory Research, 5*:159-175, 1965.

———: Auditory behavior in the human neonate: Functional properties of sound and their ontogenetic implications. *International Audiology, 8:* 34-43, 1969.

———: The development of hearing in man: An assessment of current status. *ASHA, 12*:119-123, 1970.

———: The organization of auditory behavior. *J Speech Hear Res, 13*:453-471, 1970.

———: Pediatric audiology: Shadow or substance. *Journal of Auditory Research, 11*:148-153, 1971.

Elliot, G. and Elliot, K.: Some pathological, radiological and clinical development of the human ear. *Laryngoscope, 79:*1160-1171, 1964.

Frisina, D. Measurement of hearing in children. In Jerger, J.: *Modern Developments in Audiology.* New York: Academic Press, 1973.

Froding, C.: Acoustic investigation of newborn infants. *Acta Otolaryngol, 52:*31-40, 1966.

Gesell, A. and Amatruda, C.: *Developmental Diagnosis.* New York: Paul P. Hoeber, Inc., 1947.

Griffiths, R.: *Abilities of Babies.* New York: McGraw-Hill Book Company, Inc., 1954.

Hardy, E.: Evaluation of hearing in infants and young children. In Glorig, A.: *Audiometry: Principles and Practices.* Baltimore: Williams & Wilkins Co., 1965.

Hardy, J., Dougherty, A., and Hardy, W.: Hearing responses and audiologic screening in infants. *J Pediatr, 55:*382-390, 1959.

Heron, T. and Jacobs, R.: A physiological response of the neonate to auditory stimulation. *International Audiology, 7:*41-47, 1968.

Hodgson, W.: Tests of Hearing—Birth through one year. Martin, Frederich (Ed.): *Pediatric Audiology.* Englewood Cliffs: Prentice-Hall, 1978.

Hoversten, G. and Moncur, J.: Stimuli and intensity factors in testing infants. *J Speech Hear Res, 12:*687-702, 1969.

Johansson, B., Wedenberg, E. and Westra, B.: Measurement of tone response by the human fetus. *Acta Otolaryngol, 57:*188-192, 1964.

Keith, R.W.: Impedance audiometry with neonates. *Arch Otolaryngol, 101:*376-379, 1975.

Liden, G. and Kankkunen, A.: Visual reinforcement audiometry in the management of young deaf children. *International Audiology, 8:*99-106, 1969.

Ling, D.: Response validity in auditory tests of newborn infants. *Laryngoscope, 82:*362-380, 1972.

Ling, D., Ling, A., and Doehring, D.: Stimulus, response, and observer variables in the auditory screening of newborn infants. *J Speech Hear Res, 13:*9-17, 1970.

Marge, M.: The general problem of language disabilities in children. In Irwin, J. and Marge, M.: *Principles of Childhood Language Disabilities.* New York: Appleton-Century-Crofts, 1972.

Matkin, N. and Thomas, J.: A longitudinal study of visual reinforcement audiometry. Presentation, 1975 convention, American Speech & Hearing Association.

Mencher, G. (Ed.): *Early Identification of Hearing Loss,* Basel: S. Karger, 1976.

Mendel, M.: Infant responses to recorded sounds. *J Speech Hear Res, 11:* 811-816, 1968.

Murphy, K.:   The psychophysiological maturation of auditory function. *International Audiology, 8:*46-51, 1969.

Naughton, R. and Zerlin, S.:   Basis and some diagnostic implications of electrocochleography. *Laryngoscope, 86:*475-482, 1976.

Robertson, E., Peterson, J. and Lamb, L.:   Relative impedance measurements in young children. *Arch Otolaryngol, 88:*162-168, 1968.

Seestedt, L. and Bess, F.:   Infant behavioral response to auditory stimulation.   Presentation, 1975 convention, American Speech and Hearing Association.

Suzuki, T. and Oziba, Y.:   Conditioned orientation reflex audiometry. *Arch Otolaryngol, 74:*192-198, 1961.

Taylor, D. and Mencher, G.:   Neonate response—the effect of infant state and auditory stimuli. *Arch Otolaryngol, 95:*120-124, 1972.

Thompson, G. and Weber, B.:   Response of infants and young children to behavior observation audiometry (BOA). *J Speech Hear Disord, 39:* 140-147, 1974.

Thompson, M. and Thompson, G.:   Response of infants and young children as a function of auditory stimuli and test methods. *J Speech Hear Res, 15:*699-707, 1972.

Turkewitz, G., Birch, H., and Cooper, K.:   Responsiveness to simple and complex auditory stimuli in the human newborn. *Developmental Psychobiology, 5:*7-19, 1972.

Vasiliu, D.:   L'enfant est pret a entendre meme dans la vie intrauterine, contributions sur l'embryogenese de L'oriella et la pneumatisation de la mastroide et du rocher. *International Audiology, 7:* 1968.

Waldon, E.:   Audio-reflexometry in testing hearing of very young children. *Audiology, 12:*14-20, 1973.

Chapter 10

AURAL REHABILITATION
WITH CHILDREN

Laura J. Kelly

THE PROCESS of aural rehabilitation with children is both fasci-
nating and frustrating, but it never ceases to be a challenge.
Part of the challenge arises from the need to determine the best
approach to rehabilitation for each child. Because of the large
number of variables that can affect the successful development of
language, the program needs to be as individual as possible.
Some of the factors that need to be considered include the following:

1. The time between onset and detection.
2. Age of onset of the loss.
3. The type and degree of hearing loss.
4. The presence of other handicaps.
5. Availability of services and the methodology they employ.
6. Willingness of parents to participate in the rehabilitation
   process.

All of these will affect the emphasis and the direction of the rehabilitation program.

Early Detection and Age of Onset

One of the most important factors in the success of any rehabilitation program is the early detection of the hearing impairment. If the program is to follow as closely as possible normal
auditory and language development, every day that passes without
detection means a day lost in the developmental sequence. For

example, a study by Butterfield (1968) investigated the sucking behavior of one-day-old babies when the pacifier controlled tape-recorded music; results indicated that audition affects cognition in children as young as one day old. A similar study by Eimas and others (1972) considered infant differentiation between phonemes. It seems that as early as one month, infants can perceive differences in onset time of phonemes.

These and similar studies show that from the moment of birth the auditory mechanism is delivering information to the brain; every day the infant learns more about how to use this auditory information.

It is not known at what point the effects of an impairment become irreversible, if in fact they can be reversed. Northern and Downs (1974) feel there is a point or critical period beyond which it becomes increasingly difficult for the individual to make use of certain stimuli. With the normal hearing infant it requires close to a year of audition to create the basis for the first word. More than one-half of this time is taken up with reflexive behaviors, which act to ready the verbal and auditory feedback mechanisms. The hearing impaired, then, must receive help as close to that first year as possible to make use of those reflexive patterns. Similarly, if the hearing impairment is a progressive one, or is not acquired until after certain critical periods, then the groundwork for normal development has been laid. Therapy, then, acts to maintain the skills already present and proceeds to build upon them according to the normal auditory and language sequence.

It should be pointed out that early detection needs to be followed immediately by the acquisition of appropriate amplification so that residual hearing can be put to use.

The Nature of Hearing Loss

The type and degree of hearing loss will also affect the kind of rehabilitation program and the child's prognosis. For example, if medical analysis indicates the absence of inner ear structures, a hearing aid becomes useless, and the emphasis should be placed on visual and/or tactile modes of communication. In the majority of children, however, some residual hearing is present, and through the use of appropriate amplification, it can be used. A large part of the aural rehabilitation process is to train the child to use his hearing aid to his best advantage. Some children are able to hear within a normal range with amplification. It is the clinician's job to refine that hearing, for it may be that the child hears the stimulus but does not discriminate between the sounds. Another child's impairment will be severe enough to warrant training on just knowing when important sounds have occurred.

Information can be obtained from several sources on how the child is using his hearing. The audiological report should indicate how the child does with and without the hearing aid. Parents are also a good source of information. Finally, observations of the child's behavior will demonstrate his listening skills. All of the above information needs to be taken into consideration, because it is possible for two children with similar hearing impairments to react quite differently due to factors other than the loss outlined on the audiogram (Johnson, 1978).

Often, very little information has been obtained on the nature of the impairment. The habilitation program should then take the form of diagnostic therapy. The normal process of auditory training is altered to include the use of a portable audiometer for short periods during each therapy session. Several sessions may be necessary to teach the child to use the earphones. At first this may include holding the earphone next to the child's ear while the signal is presented, and having him perform a simple task such as dropping a block into a bucket. A variety of games can be employed with the conditioning procedure to maintain the child's interest, include puzzles, building blocks, and pegboards.

The Presence of Other Handicaps

Multiply handicapped children present very special problems to the clinician. One of the main difficulties lies in testing. In the case of disorders such as mental retardation, emotional disturbance, or aphasia, many similarities exist in the behavior of speech and language, responses to sound, and inappropriate or hyperactive behaviors (Hodgson, 1969). Consequently, one disorder can mask out the presence of another for many years, resulting in misdirected therapy. The hearing impairment may be the least severe of the multiple handicaps that exist. The clinician must be prepared to work very closely with other professional personnel to plan an *overall* therapy program so that the various techniques employed by many professionals will support each other. Once again it may be necessary to use a diagnostic therapy approach to gain information about this child.

Methodology

Aural habilitation with older children will have to consider other services the child is receiving. With preschool children, the audiologist may be the only person who has contact with the family at that time and must proceed with the method most appropriate for that child and family. This will usually entail a decision between a unisensory and a multisensory approach. This decision must be made in conjunction with the parents. It is the clinician's responsibility to acquaint them with the pros and cons of the methods and discuss with them an outline of the plan chosen as well as a list of alternative services. Many parents have strong feelings about their child's education, and these need to be considered. Without parent cooperation, the habilitation process is greatly hampered.

The procedures outlined in this chapter are primarily for an auditory approach. The goal is the integration of the hearing impaired child, not just into the normal classroom but into the hearing world through a useful communication system (Hayes, 1976). The emphasis is developing the use of residual hearing to its maximum potential. Manual communication or sign language is not used. This is not to say that these procedures cannot be used in conjunction with this method. It is felt, however, that especially during the preschool years the primary focus should be placed on the auditory approach if integration into the hearing world is to be achieved successfully.

Parent Involvement

The process of language development for the hearing impaired is one that begins at birth and continues throughout the person's lifetime. For this reason, the foundation that is laid during the preschool years is of the utmost importance, for it will determine successes later on. The involvement of the family, especially the parents, in language building cannot be overemphasized. Only a small portion of the child's week will be spent in a therapy situation. The rest of the time he will be at home. Jorgensen (1970) feels parent involvement is the first factor determining whether the child will be integrated into the hearing world. Consequently, priority must be placed on helping the parents use that environment to the best advantage for their child. The following sections dealing with auditory training and language stimulation contain guidelines easily adaptable to the home or more structured therapy situations. Through counseling, demonstration, and participation, parents can become familiar with these methods and use them effectively. Though the majority of this chapter discusses the preschool child, the basic procedures are applicable to school age children as well. The clinician should always spend time talking to the parents; they are a valuable source of information and a valuable source of language and encouragement to their child. No habilitation program can reach its maximum potential unless parental guidance and cooperation are part of the total program.

Family Counseling

Following the detection of the hearing loss, the parents and family will need information if they are to fully understand the problem of hearing impairment. The habilitation process begins with the education and guidance of family members. At the initial session, the parents should be present without other family members except for the child. Northcott (1966) suggests the clinician listen carefully and observe the way in which the parents deal with their child. What are the parents' feelings about hearing loss. Has this changed their attitude toward their child? How does the child deal with emotion? Does he use his voice spontaneously or does he rely totally on gestures? This information can be useful in determining family attitudes.

Northcott (1966) also suggests that the parents keep a notebook about the child's reactions to sounds and his use of voice at home. The parents will then have a yardstick by which to measure progress. It will also give the clinician a chronicle of the parents' view of the child's behavior in the home.

The next two sessions should include as many family members as are able to attend and any older children who are able to understand. Other interested persons, such as a regular babysitter, may also benefit by attending these sessions. Care should be taken, however, to prevent the group from becoming too large or the parents from feeling stifled in asking questions. The atmosphere needs to be relaxed and open so that concerns can be discussed as easily as possible. Sometimes individual sessions with husband and wife can also afford an opportunity for the expression of feelings or asking specific questions in cases where one or the other is dominating the discussion.

The best way to alleviate the fears and myths about hearing loss is through education. Parents should be told what hearing loss is, the simple anatomy and how the mechanisms work, how hearing is tested, what an audiogram shows, and which sounds can and cannot be heard by the child. Whenever possible, these explanations should be accompanied by diagrams and demonstrations.

Every hearing impaired child for whom amplification is appropriate should wear his aid as often and as long as possible. This may involve helping the parents gradually increase the the length of time each day the aid is worn. A mark can be placed on the volume control of the hearing aid to ensure it will not be turned up beyond a particular point. This will prevent the amplification from becoming annoying to the new hearing aid wearer. If the hearing aid is worn during quiet activities such as coloring and reading, it will also help to ease the child into listening with the aid. The periods when the aid is worn should be rewarded with praise and attention.

A problem that often arises is concern about placement of a body type of hearing aid. The first reaction is to place it underneath clothing, either to hide it from view or to try to protect it. Parents should know the pros and cons of various aid positionings and be given suggestions to help alleviate problems such as excessive clothing noise. For example, pockets that button shut placed near the shoulder can be added to children's clothing relatively easy. Back placement is sometimes advisable with children who are crawling.

Parents with children entering school for the first time may be concerned about the other children's acceptance of the hearing aid. They can be assured that there may be a burst of curiosity during the first days and maybe even a little jealous over this strange device, but generally the hearing aid is accepted without problems (Stassens, 1973).

For children using an amplification system, a comprehensive hearing aid orientation should be conducted. With preschoolers the parents will obviously be responsible for the aid's care; however, the child should be encouraged to take on various responsibilities as soon as he is able. Most children adjust to the task of wearing a hearing aid readily. It is not uncommon for the young child to bring the aid to his parents as soon as something becomes detached, lost, or when the aid is not amplifying.

The hearing aid orientation should cover the operation, care, and maintenance of a hearing aid. It should be emphasized that a hearing aid is only a tool and, as such, will not allow the child to hear everything we do. Consequently, limitations should be spelled out to avoid the expectation of "perfect" hearing. At the same time, parents need to understand that, however imperfect these devices are, they are now acting as their child's ears. As such they will be in use continually, and proper maintenance is essential. To make sure that parents feel comfortable with daily maintenance and troubleshooting techniques, it is best to guide them through step-by-step procedures. A sample troubleshooting guide has been included in Appendix A.

Inform the parents that it is advisable to have the child's hearing and hearing aid retested at regular intervals. During the preschool years, the time lapse should not be over one year. If the child is prone to ear infections and if the aid is used roughly, the checks need to be more frequent. Advise the parents to bring the child in if they notice a sudden change in his response to sound. His residual hearing is precious to him, and it will be well worth the effort to preserve it.

Lastly, discuss with them the services that are available in education, information, and funding. If the state has laws relating to the education of the handicapped, they should be explained along with the rights of the handicapped under the law. A list of agencies that can be helpful to parents has been included at the end of this chapter.

It should never be assumed that parents are already familiar with this information. All too often no one has bothered to explain basic information to them. Parents have a right and a need to know about their child's hearing impairment if they are to work as an effective part of the habilitation process.

The Auditory Training Process

The auditory training program can begin immediately following detection of the hearing loss even though the hearing aid has not yet been fitted. Even infants may have auditory training. In a study of three hearing impaired infants, Mavilya (1972) demonstrated that the babbling behavior of these infants increased to a peak as did normal infants, but instead of proceeding into the stage of imitation, the hearing impaired children's vocalizations declined sharply. For this reason it is important to begin talking to the child even at this early stage. Downs (1968) feels that speaking to the child during the babbling stage helps to develop normal intonation patterns. Rehabilitation with infants need not include formal sessions; just talking to the child helps to create a pleasant listening atmosphere. Many audiologists, including Northcott (1967), advocate the use of normal daily activities, including bathing, changing, and playing with the infant. During these activities, listening and language are stimulated.

At this point a differentiation needs to be drawn between hearing and listening. Through the use of hearing aids, the hearing impaired child is able to hear, but is he listening? Most likely not, and if he is not, he is not making use of the sound as an important source of information. To help parents understand this, a simple exercise can be conducted. Have them take a piece of paper and walk into several different rooms in their home, including kitchen, living room bedroom, and bathroom. In each room have them list ten sounds they hear. Parents are usually surprised at how many sounds they take for granted, and they also begin to realize how much information in their environment is transmitted via nonverbal sounds.

To develop sound awareness, almost any sound can be used. It is a good idea, however, to follow some simple criteria at first. The sound should be one you can control and initially needs to be loud enough to draw the child's attention to it. Later, emphasis can be placed on loud-soft discrimination. In the meantime, make sure he can hear it clearly. Along with control, consider whether the sound can be repeated. You will probably want to have several trials with the same sound each day. The stimuli should also be interesting to the child; for example, toy vacuum cleaners, hair dryers, pots and pans all hold fascination for children. These objects also have the advantage of being a meaningful part of the child's daily routine. Many times a sound will be more interesting if it makes something happen. An example of such a toy is the jack-in-the-box where the music precedes the box opening.

In the initial stages of sound awareness, visual as well as auditory modes should be used so the interest is maintained and an association is developed between the sound and the object that makes it. Consequently, the child's attention is drawn to the object to ready him for the sound production. When the sound is produced, act excited and happy. The Bill Wilkerson Hearing and Speech Center (1976) made the following suggestions. Show the child that listening is enjoyable and you are involved by saying, "Listen, I hear the sound" or "I hear the . . . ." Placing the hands by the ears when the sound is produced can help to draw attention to the primary locus of the stimuli. Repeating the sound with your voice following the presentation encourages imitation by the child to respond to your actions. A pause following your imitation gives him the opportunity to join in.

Following the establishment of a consistent gross-sound discrimination, finer differentiations can begin as in the association of a sound with a particular object and the discrimination between two sounds. This can be done informally in the home as in differentiating between the water running and the dishes during cleanup, or it may be done in games during therapy. Choices should be limited at first to two items and then increased as discrimination ability improves. The items can be hidden in a large box, under a table, behind the back, or the child can close his eyes.

Throughout this time, the child's attention should be drawn to loud sounds outside of the task being performed; this is especially true in the home. For example, if a car horn is honked, say, "Listen, I hear it," put the hands by the ears, and take the child to the window to look at what is making the noise. In this way an awareness to sound outside the immediate area is encouraged.

When working with older children, gross-sound discrimination can also be useful, especially when environmental sounds are used (Sanders, 1971). An informal evaluation of these skills is helpful before proceeding on to more difficult tasks of speech discrimination.

Speech discrimination involves more than telling the difference between *s* and *t*. For this reason, speech discrimination can also be conducted with very young children. Hudgins and Numbers (1942) cited several factors, which they called the prerequisites for intelligible speech: general factors such as speech rhythm, accentuation, grouping and phrasing, voice quality, and intonation. Grouping and phrasing can be developed through listening to the speech of others. Rhythm, voice quality, accentuation, and intonation can be facilitated through means such as music, clapping and rhythm games, accompanying activities with rhymes and songs, and demonstrating the variations in the teacher's own voice. Older children can be asked to differentiate between types of phrases such as a statement, a question, and an exclamation of surprise. Some examples of activities to use with children have been included in Appendix B.

Auditory training is fundamental to the aural habilitation process. Many of the finer aspects of auditory training are developed through working with speech, but returning to the basics to reemphasize skills can be very helpful, especially with younger children when they begin to speak and attend to the speech of others. Parents become involved with working on the development of language to the exclusion of auditory training. They should be reminded that continuing to reinforce auditory awareness to sound will train the child to make use of all sounds for information and not just speech. Vorce (1971) reaffirms this continued training of listening skills with older children, stating that listening should become a part of educational settings by using a wide range of situations and experiences.

Language Stimulation

Every situation is a language learning situation for the hearing impaired. The objects around us, which we take for granted in our lives, all have names and uses that are new and interesting to children. They can be tasted, touched, smelled, manipulated, experienced and, most importantly, talked about. The role of clinician or parent becomes that of a model to present as much stimulation and as many correct examples as can be fitted into each day. Many parents are intimidated by this role. It is important to reassure them that they are probably already doing most of the same things that are done in a therapy setting; with guidance, they can learn to use them more effectively.

To begin speech and language training, speak in a normal tone of voice as close to the child's level as possible (Ewing and Ewing, 1964). If you are standing above him while he is on the floor, not only will the sound stimuli be misdirected, but he will also lose valuable clues from your gestures, facial expression, and speech reading. Through *natural* gestures, intonation, and facial expression, show your own enthusiasm for the activity. Do not, however, make him look at you while you talk, but make it easier for him to use the clues should he choose to (McConnell, 1971). By being at his level, you are also demonstrating a personal interest in him and what he is doing, thus helping to maintain his attention.

Activities should be interesting to the child. To help make them so, plan to have the child take an active part. Remember that things that are commonplace for you are new to the child.

An example of a household job of which children never seem to tire is washing dishes. They love the water, and it provides a great opportunity to talk about household items such as knives, forks, dishes, pots and pans. A similar activity can make use of a small snack with cleanup afterward. Remember to check with parents before any food or drinks are given to children. The children may have an allergy or be on a special diet.

Talk about what you are doing each moment. It may be obvious to *you*, but the hearing impaired child may not possess the words for describing the activity; use the name of an object individually and then place it into a sentence. This will provide an association between the object and the word and also give a model of its association to other words.

For the child who does not yet use spoken words, the sentences should be short and simple (McConnell, 1971). Occasionally, place the child's own thoughts and feelings into words. For example, if the child has cut his finger, "Mommy, my finger hurts!!" (Lillie, 1976). This not only provides him with an example of how to express what he feels, it also shows him you understand. In expressing his thoughts separately, you identify him as an individual in his own right, which promotes a solid self-concept. Most importantly, repeat everything over and over again. If you think you said the word a hundred times, place it in countless sentences, say it another thousand. It is through constant exposure that language is learned. As an example of the importance of imitation in language development, Sweeney (1973) reports the case of a six-week-old infant who, following exposure to bird calls for four days, began imitating those sounds. Her birdlike vocalizations increased when the birds were present and eventually disappeared after removal of the pets.

To encourage a child to make sounds, reinforcement is needed for all his attempts (Downs, 1967). This can be done through praise and by imitating the sounds after the child. Invent sounds to accompany his movements and games so that listening and participation will be interesting. Repetition of nonsense sounds in rhythmic patterns of varying intonation will also help him to develop inflection and refined listening skills.

When the child is already using words, the process of auditory training becomes one of reinforcement of existing vocabulary and expansion to more difficult structures. Single words he uses should be placed into sentences and incomplete phrases converted into whole ones. All attempts should be reinforced and approved, but if he uses incorrect language, the correct models should be provided. By your use of new words along with the old, vocabulary will be increased to his and by increasing the complexity of your sentence form, alternatives to his way of expressing ideas are presented (Lillie, 1976).

Examples of how not to talk to the child will be discussed. There are times when silence can provide the best therapy. Schwarzberg (1975) feels that to want to say anything the child must have a good concept of self; once this is achieved, the child will naturally wish to communicate his feelings about himself and the world. If he is to make the attempt and then continue to communicate, the child has to have a good receiver. This entails giving *him* the chance to make the noise and being genuinely interested in what he has to say and what he is doing. Schwartzberg states that this approach pays off in more than just reinforcement of language, it will also improve listening skills. Learning is facilitated by demonstration, and if an example of interested listening is presented, the child will imitate it. A young child can also be discouraged from talking if he is continually asked to name objects or repeat words. This is an easy habit for parents to develop. As stated earlier, when incorrect language or pronunciation is used, the correct model should be provided, but to insist that the child repeat it until it is correct is frustrating for the child. He may not have developed his discrimination skills to the point of being able to hear his mistake.

When planning the actual (re)habilitation session, remain as flexible as possible while still maintaining control. There will be many times when the child will not be the least bit interested in what you have planned for the day. Forcing him to participate will only frustrate both of you, so take a moment and find out what he wants to do. By allowing decisions of this nature, self-expression is encouraged. You can still control the direction and emphasis of what is occurring. To help in these situations, it is also wise to keep in reserve one activity that is always a favorite with that particular child. If you must move the session into the bathroom so you can use the sink for washing play dishes, then do so and take advantage of the real situation. There is nothing worse than spending an hour with a fussy, disinterested four-year-old. Another common pitfall is running out of material; this happens quite often with children. It may be that on a particular day you can spend the whole time on one or two activities through which he is continually fascinated; the next session, ten activities may not be enough. A good rule of thumb is to always plan too much material. More often than not, it will not be too much at all. If you do not use all of the material, it can always be carried over to the next session.

The actual format of the therapy session might follow this outline:

1. Discuss with the parents the previous week's assignments— both the successful aspects and the problems.
2. Explain the emphasis for that day's session, such as practice with repetition.
3. Proceed with an activity and begin to gradually include the parents.
4. Allow time at the end of the session to assess what was good and what needs some improvement.
4. Give them a homework assignment that is similar, if possible, to the clinic activity. This will facilitate carryover.

The excerpt below demonstrates an activity in the therapy session. The phrases are listed as examples and so do not contain the pauses that would normally occur. This activity included use of unbreakable kitchen utensils such as silverware, measuring cups, plastic or metal bowls, etc. and a sink.

> Here it is, Steve. It's a big sink. Turn on the water. Do you hear the water? SSSS. The water is loud. The water makes a lot of noise. The water is cold. Feel the water. Turn the water off, Steve. Do you see the water splash? Is the spoon in the water? The spoon is under the water. Whoops, there goes the water! The water has gone down the drain.

Many key words can be substituted in the activity. Another activity is giving a doll a bath and discussing body parts.

The preceding example demonstrates that there is no real magic to language stimulation with children. A concentrated effort to provide all kinds of experience in extra-large doses may be defined as language stimulation. A hearing impaired child is normal in every way except for his hearing sensitivity. He is a part of the family and should be as much involved with all the activities as any member of the family (Magner, 1971).

Many times it is advisable to place the child in a normal nursery school so that he can be exposed to the flow of language from other children. Northcott (1971) suggested that supplemental rehabilitative help may be beneficial and provides extra language stimulation and reinforcement of his experiences. Actual structured sessions with some drill are applicable when the child has begun to use his speech spontaneously in phrases (Magner, 1971).

A Final Note

Aural habilitation can be a relaxed and enjoyable experience for those involved. In creating such an atmosphere, communication and the active exchange of information are facilitated. When communication becomes tedious and boring, the effort to make it work may disappear along with the will to communicate. Establishing a friendly professional atmosphere is possible; when this is achieved, the clinician can learn equally from the client.

References

Butterfield, E.C.: "An extended version of modification of sucking with auditory feedback." Working Paper #43, Bureau of Child Research Laboratory, Childrens Rehabilitation Unit, University of Kansas Medical Center, 1968.

Downs, M.P.: "Early identification and Principles of Management." ICOED, Washington, D.C., Alexander Graham Bell Association for the Deaf 74688, 1967.

Downs, M.P.: "Identification and training of Deaf Children: Birth to One Year." *Volta Review:* 70:154-158, 1968.

Eimas, P.D., Siqueland, E.R., Jusczk, P., and Vigorit, J.: "Speech Perception in Infants." *Science, 171:*303, 1972.

Ewing, A. and Ewing, C.: *Teaching Deaf Children to Talk.* Manchester, England: Manchester Press, 105-141, 1964.

Hayes, D.M.: "An Auditory-Oral Program." Parents of the Auditory-Oral Program in the Madison Public Schools, Madison, Wisconsin, February, 1976.

Hodgson, W.R.: "Misdiagnosis of Children with Hearing Loss." *The Journal of School Health, 398:*510-515 (1969).

Hudgins, C.V. and Numbers, F.C.: "An Investigation of the Intelligibility of the Speech of the Deaf." *Genetic and Psychology Monograph, 25,* 289-392, 1972.

Johnson, E.W.: "Let's Look at the Child, Not the Audiogram," *The Hearing Impaired Child in the Regular Classroom.* W. H. Northcott (Ed.), Washington, D.C., Alexander Graham Bell Association for the Deaf, 18-23, 1973.

Jorgensen, I.S.: "Special Education in Denmark." *Det Danske Selskb,* 1970.

Lillie, S.M.: Talking Language Development Programs. Bill Wilkerson Hearing and Speech Center, 1114 19th Avenue, South, Nashville, Tennessee, 1976.

Magner, M.E.: "Techniques of Teaching." *Speech for the Deaf Child: Knowledge and Use.* L.E. Conner (Ed.), Washington, D.C., Alexander Graham Bell Association for the Deaf, 245-264, 1971.

Mavilya, M.: "Spontaneous Vocalization and Babbling in the Hearing Impaired Infant," *International Symposium on Speech Communication Ability and Profound Deafness.* G. Fant (Ed.): Ann Arbor, Michigan, Edwards Brothers, Inc., 1972.

McConnell, F.: "The Psychology of Communication," *Speech for the Deaf Child: Knowledge and Use.* L.E. Conner (Ed.), Washington, D.C., Alexander Graham Bell Association for the Deaf, 170-182, 1971.

Northcott, W.N.: "Counseling Parents of Pre-school Hearing Impaired." *ICOED,* 424-442, 1967.

Northcott, W.N.: "Infant Education and Home Training," *Speech for the Deaf Child: Knowledge and Use.* L.E. Conner (Ed.), Washington, D.C., Alexander Graham Bell Association for the Deaf, 311-334, 1971.

Northcott, W.: "Language Development Through Parent Counseling and Guidance." *Volta Review, 68:*356-360, 1966.

Northern, J.L. and Downs, M.: *Hearing in Children.* Baltimore, Maryland, The Williams and Wilkins Company, 1974.

Sanders, D.A.: *Aural Rehabilitation,* Englewood Cliffs, New Jersey, Prentice-Hall, Inc., 1971.

Schwartzberg, J.G.: "Parent Effectiveness: Helping Your Child Achieve Better Langauage." *The Volta Review, 17:*296-302, 1975.

Simmons, A.A.: "Language Growth for the Pre-Nursery Deaf Child." *Volta*

Review, 68:201-205, 1966.

Stassens, R.A.: "I Have One in My Class Who's Wearing Hearing Aids." *The Hearing Impaired Child in the Regular Classroom.* W.H. Northcott (Ed.), Washington, D.C., Alexander Graham Bell Association for the Deaf, 24-31, 1973.

Sweeney, S.: "The Importance of Imitation in the Early Stages of Speech Acquisition: A Case Report." *J Speech Hear Dirosd, 38*:490-494, 1973.

Vorce, E.: "Speech Curriculum," *Speech for the Deaf Child: Knowledge and Use,* L.E. Connor (Ed.), Washington, D.C., Alexander Graham Bell Association for the Deaf, 221-244, 1971.

Wilkerson, Bill Hearing and Speech Center. "First Listening Lessons for Very Young Deaf Children," Video Tape, Directors: F. McConnell and K. Horton, 1976.

TROUBLESHOOTING GUIDE

Daily Hearing Aid Check:
1. Check the batteries and place it in the hearing aid case, matching the (+) and (−).
2. Turn the hearing aid to *mic* and/or *on*.
3. Place the earmold to your ear. Is it amplifying your voice? If there are other noises present, such as clicking, check the section in troubleshooting, below.
4. Turn the volume control up slowly. Is your voice getting louder? Good!
5. With a body type of aid, twist the cord gently between your fingers. Does the sound turn on and off? (If so, change to a new cord.)
6. Remove the batteries from the aid every night. In very humid weather, put the aid in a dehumidifying bag overnight.

Troubleshooting

If you can't hear any sound coming from the hearing aid—
1. Is the battery in the case properly? Check to see if the (+) on the battery is matched with (+) on the case.
2. Is the hearing aid turned to *mic* and/or *on?*
3. Is the cord plugged securely into the case and receiver?

If the sound keeps going on and off—
1. Is the battery corroded? If you see a little corrosion on the battery ends, rub them with a pencil eraser. Be sure to use the battery tester to recheck the battery.
2. Is the cord damaged? While listening to the hearing aid, squeeze and jiggle the cord a little. If the sound goes off

and on, change cords.

3. Is the cord plugged securely into the receiver and hearing aid case?
4. Check the receiver; it may be cracked.

If the volume is weak—

1. Check the battery with the battery tester. If it registers "weak" or "dead," change the battery.

If you hear a feedback squeal—

1. Check your child's earmolds. Make sure they are fitting in the ears properly. You may need new earmolds. Children outgrow earmolds frequently between the ages of 1 to 5.
2. Check the receiver nozzle to see if it is worn. Be sure to use the "receiver savers."

If you hear muffled or distorted sound—

1. The microphone screen may be dirty. Brush it off with a soft brush. DO NOT try to open the case; it may void your warranty.
2. Did the hearing aid get wet? If so, put it in a dehumidifier bag or in a hair dryer bonnet set on COOL. If the air is warm or hot, it could ruin the hearing aid.
3. Check the earmold; it may be plugged with ear wax or worn (cracks in it). Wash earmolds regularly with lukewarm, sudsy water. Remove all wax from canal portion. Be sure the earmold is completely dry before snapping it to the receiver.

INFORMATION FOR HOME AND FAMILY

Activities for the home or home setting with preschool children.

Around the House

1. make a cake
2. make jello
3. wash dishes
4. make cookies
5. wash the sink
6. talk on the telephone
7. make the bed
8. wash windows
9. wax/dust furniture
10. vacuum carpeting
11. take a bath
12. fold clothes
13. dressing or changing clothes
14. make a doll dress
15. shine shoes
16. rearrange furniture
17. iron clothes
18. put socks together
19. wash doll clothing
20. read a book together
21. cut out pictures
22. Play-Doh®
23. finger paint
24. color
25. set the table
26. have a snack
27. look at family pictures
28. a "sound walk" around the house to listen to the sound maker, i.e. disposal, vacuum cleaner, TV, hair dryer, mixer.

Outdoors

1. playing in the sandbox
2. digging in dirt
3. making mud pies
4. riding a bike
5. pick or plant flowers
6. sliding
7. climbing—hills, trees, jungle gym
8. swimming
9. playing with hose or sprinkler
10. fly a kite
11. go fishing
12. go for a walk
13. cut the grass
14. swinging

15. wash the car
16. trim the hedges
17. water the grass
18. have a picnic
19. rake leaves

20. feed the birds
21. take a walk
22. look at bugs
23. sweep the walk
24. hang clothes out to dry

Seasonal

1. decorate a Christmas tree
2. make Christmas cards
3. make valentines
4. carve a pumpkin
5. boil and color eggs for Easter

6. wrapping Christmas presents
7. make a Thanksgiving pie
8. make a snowman and come in for hot chocolate
9. make an Easter breakfast
10. have a birthday party

Miscellaneous

1. blowing bubbles
2. shopping for clothes, groceries
3. riding in a car
4. going to a restaurant or ice cream parlor

5. going to the airport
6. going to a railroad station
7. have a carnival
8. go to the zoo
9. have a parade
10. visit the grandparents

Periodically, pictures can be taken or drawn of activities and placed into the child's notebook. It not only gives a record of happenings, but becomes an activity in itself and a constant review of previous vocabulary.

Suggested Family Counseling Outline

Session I.   Family Attitudes

A. General Discussion of family life while making observations.
B. Hearing loss
 1. attitudes towards hearing loss in general.
 2. attitudes towards hearing aid.
C. Parents feelings toward child's loss
 1. relationship to other people
 2. educating prospects
D. Sibling feeling toward child's loss
E. Compiling notebook of progress

Session II. What Is Hearing Loss?
A. Anatomy
   1. Outer
   2. Middle Ear
      a. tympanic membrane
      b. ossicular chain
      c. eustachian tube
      d. how the system transfers sound
   3. Inner Ear
      a. bony shell
      b. fluid filled
      c. action of hair cells
      d. activates nerves to brain
B. Hearing Testing
   1. Pure tones
   2. Speech Audiometry
   3. Impedance
   4. What each tells us
C. The Audiogram
   1. What it means
   2. Explanation of child's own hearing tests
D. The Hearing Aid
   1. Components
      a. microphone
      b. receiver
      c. on-off and tone controls
      d. telephone
   2. Operations
E. Care and Maintenance
   1. Daily check
   2. Troubleshooting
F. Wearing the aid
   1. Adjusting to the aid
   2. Position of aid
      a. harness on back
      b. harness on front
      c. pockets in clothes

G. Periodic Evaluations
1. Hearing
2. Hearing Aid

Session III.   Services Available

A. Sources of Information
B. Sources of Funding

SOURCES OF INFORMATION FOR PARENTS

Alexander Graham Bell
Association for the Deaf, Inc.
Volta Bureau
1537 35th Street N.W.
Washington, D.C. 20007

American Speech, Language & Hearing Association
10801 Rockville Pike
Rockville, Maryland 20852

Bill Wilkerson Hearing & Speech Center
1114 19th Avenue, South
Nashville, Tennessee 37212

John Tracy Clinic
806 West Adams Boulevard
Los Angeles, California 90007

Lexington School for the Deaf
30th Avenue and 75th Street
Jackson Heights, NY 11370

AUTHOR INDEX

Chomsky, N., 3, 36
Clark, E.V., 25, 36, 44, 61
Clayborne, D., 141, 167
Coleman, R.F., 232, 239, 240, 250
Collins, N., 166, 167
Conner, L.E., 304
Cook, P., 69, 89
Cooper, E.B., 197
Cooper, K., 288
Costello, J., 121, 124, 125, 140, 158, 168
Coursia, D., 286
Crystal, D., 59, 61
Cunningham, R., 149
Curlee, R.F., 207, 209, 219, 220
Curtis, J.F., 219, 221, 250, 251

D

Dale, P.A., 28, 36
Dallos, P., 285, 286
Damsté, P.H., 222, 251, 226
Daniloff, R.G., 13, 38
Darley, F.L., 13, 39, 137, 219, 241
Davis, D.M., 184, 219
Davis, H., 275, 276
Davis, S., 122, 154, 156, 163, 170, 178
Delbridge, 168
Demmitt, K., 169
DeVilliers, J.G., 11, 36, 52, 61
DeVilliers, P.A., 11, 36, 52, 61
Dickson, S., 171, 220, 240, 251
Diedrich, W.M., 144, 145, 147, 162, 168, 177, 178
Dingwall, W.O., 38
Dirks, D.D., 256, 258, 276
Doehring, D., 287
Dougherty, A., 287
Downing, L., 90
Downs, M., 286, 290, 296, 300, 304
Dublinski, S., 139, 141, 145, 168
Duguay, M., 226, 252
Dunn, L.M., 21, 36, 59, 61, 104, 116
121, 138, 168
Dwornicka, B., 279, 286

E

Edney, C.W., 219
Egan, J.P., 268, 276
Eggermont, J., 285, 286
Egland, G.O., 190, 219

Eimas, P.D., 290, 303
Eisenberg, R., 279, 286, 280
Eisenson, J., 121, 153, 168, 190, 219, 220
Eldert, E., 276
Elliot, G., 279, 286
Elliot, K., 279, 286
Emerick, L., 8, 36
Emge, M.E., 223, 251
Engelmann, S., 59, 61
Engmann, D., 125, 169
Erickson, R.L., 200
Ervin, S.M., 27, 38
Escalona, C., 286
Eurich, K., 149
Ewing, A., 299, 304
Ewing, C., 299, 304

F

Fairbanks, G., 105, 116, 226, 231, 251, 268, 276
Fairchild, L., 145, 168
Falk, A., 64, 68, 90
Fant, G., 304
Feldman, C.F., 43, 61
Ferguson, C.A., 38
Filter, M.D., 223, 224, 229, 235, 236, 242, 250, 251
Fletcher, P., 59, 61
Flowers, A., 168
Foster, R., 22, 36
Fraser, C., 17, 18, 23, 27, 36, 46, 61
Freeman, F.J., 214
Frisina, D., 282, 287
Fristoe, M., 13, 36, 168
Froding, C., 287
Frohman, A., 91
Furst, L.C., 214, 220

G

Gallagher, T.M., 23, 38
Garmen, M., 59, 61
Gerber, A., 140, 168
Gesell, A., 281, 287
Gidden, J., 22, 36, 116
Glorig, A., 287
Gluksberg, S., 31, 36
Goda, S., 161, 163, 168
Goetzinger, C., 269, 276, 270
Goldiamond, I., 207, 219

SUBJECT INDEX